PSYCHOLOGICAL
WAR
ON
FAT

Franklin D. Cordell, Ph.D.
and
Gale R. Giebler, Ph.D.

Argus Communications
Allen, Texas 75002 U.S.A.

Cover design by Gene Tarpey
Illustrations by George Hamblin

FIRST EDITION

© Argus Communications 1977

Printed in the United States of America.

ARGUS COMMUNICATIONS
A Division of DLM, Inc.
One DLM Park
Allen, Texas 75002 U.S.A.

International Standard Book Number: 0-913592-90-0
Library of Congress Number: 77-86464

0 9 8 7 6 5 4 3

To our families
To Louise and Franklin
To Karen, John, and Bill

ABOUT THE AUTHORS

Coauthor of the popular *Am I OK?*, Franklin D. Cordell, Ph.D. has conducted numerous workshops in personal growth. In attacking excess weight he combines his extensive scholarly knowledge with firsthand experience of people and their problems.

A popular lecturer, Gale R. Giebler, Ph.D. is a clinical psychologist and counselor at the University of Northern Colorado Counseling Center. Dr. Giebler has led successful weight loss groups for several years.

Both authors have a personal interest in weight control. Using the strategies described in *Psychological War on Fat,* Dr. Cordell lost sixty pounds and Dr. Giebler thirty-five pounds.

CONTENTS

INTRODUCTION

A psychological war on fat? Isn't that going just a little too far? Can such a thing succeed?

No, it is not going too far. And yes, it is a very winnable war. This victory will change your habits, your attitudes, and your body. We know. The authors are veterans of that war.

Recent research confirms what every overweight person already knows: that being overweight is tied not only to our eating habits but also to our patterns of feeling, our assertiveness or lack of it, and our self-identity. Better yet, psychology shows us how to change our feelings of discouragement and our troublesome grazing habits, and how to enlist the help of friends in maintaining motivation.

Research from other disciplines shows us the mechanics of how to achieve a quick weight loss, and the psychological approach presented in this book adds two essential elements: (1) how to keep losing weight and (2) how to maintain an ideal weight.

Once you understand the principles underlying them, the skills are easily learned. And when applied, these skills can change your weight, your habits, and your emotional life for the better.

VISUALIZE SUCCESS

Visualize yourself on a morning sometime in the future. You wake up with a new sense of self-acceptance and self-love. As you get out of bed, you savor the morning air. Life seems precious now. These feelings are rather new to you. They replace those old feelings—feelings that you do not even like to think about anymore. You have a feeling of lightness and confidence. Think of it. A lot of things have happened to you lately.

Where did this confidence come from? As you look back, you cannot put your finger on any one thing. Rather, a series of things come to mind. Maybe it was the first time you fully realized that you were regularly losing weight because you were fully in control of your feelings about food and dieting. Maybe it was the first time you bought some new clothing and realized that you were approaching your weight-loss goal. Maybe it was when you recognized that there was a beautiful body hidden inside that shroud of fat you had carried

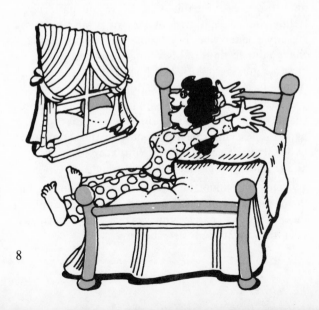

around for so long. Maybe it was the first time you were really assertive and asked for something you really wanted and needed, and you were not rejected for so doing.

Well, confidence is one thing, but there were a lot of other things. One of the things you liked most was the new vitality that came with your weight loss—the feeling of your body as it firmed up and became responsive to your commands. What a feeling of freedom came with that vitality!

One of the really beautiful consequences of your personal growth was the new set of relationships you created with other people. Your friendship was no longer tied to being a clown who had to continually apologize for who you were. Now it became based in a respect and love that derived from your newly found self-respect and self-love.

How could all that have been achieved without long periods of self-deprivation and self-punishment? Now that you understand where feelings come from, it is

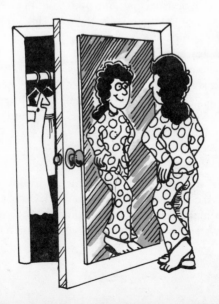

hard to see how you believed that such self-deprivation was necessary. What a sense of power to understand that you are in charge of your feelings and that feelings are not imposed upon you by a capricious and impersonal reality.

Look in the mirror just one more time. Are those sags and bulges still gone? Yes, they are! Isn't that wonderful?

YOU CAN BREAK OUT OF THE CYCLE

You *can* be free of the driving feelings of embarrassment and self-consciousness that plague you and most overweight people. You *can* experience the pure joy of living in a new, healthy, and attractive body. And you *do not* have to live with eternal dieting and feelings of deprivation for the rest of your life.

Psychology shows that there are some relatively simple ways to break out of those self-defeating cycles. This book presents those ways in a simple, easy-to-follow program. This is not a book about dieting in the normal sense, but rather a manual that shows you how to repattern your feelings and your thinking, and how to create new habits to solve the overweight problem once and for all.

Upon learning to practice the techniques in this book, you can drop those feelings of frustration and discouragement, and experience delightful new feelings about yourself. In so doing, you will lose weight naturally and keep it off without feelings of deprivation. So stop kicking yourself!

PROGRAM ORGANIZATION

There are four main sections to this book, which parallel the goals of this program. Part 1 is organized to help make sense of your feelings and behaviors. Step-by-step directions will help you achieve a healthier attitude and a lasting weight loss. This section of the book is intended to answer such questions as: Why do I feel doomed by fate to be overweight? How can I develop the self-discipline and the motivation needed to lose weight? Why do I seem to "not care" at certain times? How can I deal with discouragement? How can I repattern my feelings so as to experience the joy of being free from frustration, discouragement, and self-hate?

Part 2, on behavior modification, will help you become more aware of your inappropriate eating habits and show you some ways to change them. As you well know, even the best intentions and the best efforts to control weight are sometimes sabotaged by one's own unconscious and destructive eating habits. Psychological insights will help you become aware of your destructive eating habits and teach you how to change them in a few short weeks. This section of the book will answer such questions as: How are habits

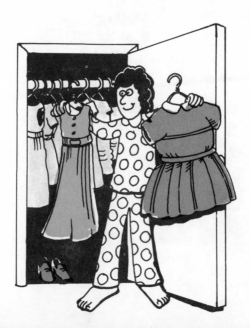

11

formed? How can I change my eating habits so that I can keep weight off? How can I change my tendency to go on eating binges?

Part 3 shows you how to build helpful relationships with other people. Overweight people often need the approval and support of others but do not know how to ask for it. So their efforts are often frustrated before they even get started. This section answers such questions as: How can I be more assertive? Should I join a weight-loss group? How do I ask for the help I need? How can I deal with people who seem to resist my efforts to change?

Part 4 provides a simple, easily understood explanation of the basic nutritional, dieting, and calorie-counting facts needed to lose weight for a lifetime.

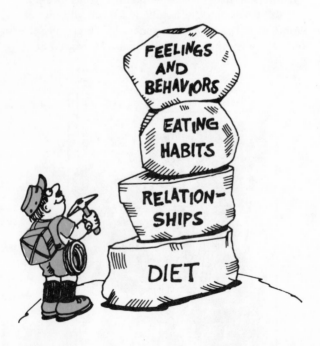

PART ONE

FEELINGS AND WEIGHT CONTROL

This section of the book deals with the feelings about self and about food and dieting that are so important in achieving a happier, more persistent approach to weight loss. In the last ten years enormous strides have been made in the development of ways to help people understand and control feelings.

After working with over one thousand obese patients at the Dietary Rehabilitation Clinic of Duke University, Gerard Musante argued that treatment must include work with the beliefs and feelings of the obese patient. The Stanford Eating Disorders Clinic programs include a component on beliefs.

It seems science is finally learning what fat people have always known: the business of being fat is a vicious circle of discouragement and eating.

victory awaits you

Jog.
Count calories.
Take miracle pills.
Suffer high-protein constipation.
Endure low-carbohydrate headaches.
Eat grapefruit and eggs three times a day.
Join the latest weight-loss group.
Fight the endless battles of the diet revolution.

Will anything work? Yes. Recent scientific findings combined into a personally tailored program can enable you to control your weight. More than that, the skills and self-assurance gained in such a program set the stage for a generally happier and healthier life.

WEIGHT CONTROL AND PERSONAL GROWTH

Have you ever wondered at the confidence, joy, vitality, friendliness, productivity, and openness that some people seem to experience? They seem to be constantly in love with life—not a blind, simple-minded love of life, but a feet-on-the-ground, life-is-an-exciting-adventure love of life. Such people are easily loved and accepted because they are so physically and socially attractive. They seem to have a kind of magnetism. Their basically healthy personalities seem to be self-sustaining. They feel good and are not driven by overpowering needs; they can act in ways that make good things happen. They get all the attention and stimulation they need because they behave in ways that make them attractive to others. In a way it is a cycle. Just as the rich get richer, the healthy get healthier. When we get our lives running in the right way, we seem to build up momentum.

Abraham Maslow explored the idea of self-actualization and found that only about one percent of the population approached the realization of their basic potential for being fully human and fully alive. It is bad news that so small a percentage achieve self-actualization, but good news that we all have the potential. Learning to control our weight is a big step toward self-actualization.

If we all have the potential to be self-actualizing, why the differences among people? Why do some people get into such a positive life-style, while most of the rest of us get sidetracked? In general, the answer is simple.

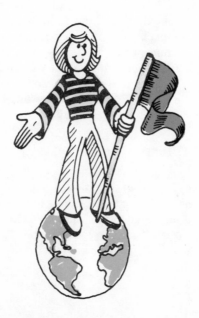

We all learn ways of solving life problems, satisfying needs, and completing life tasks. These ways of solving problems are partly conscious, partly unconscious ways of dealing with life. Some of these ways work well. For instance, if we learn to deal with anxiety and worry by getting to the cause of it, we can root out the cause and regain our balance. Other ways work well only in the short run. For instance, the habit of eating to deal with the depression of being overweight only deals with the problem temporarily. In the long run this strategy does not work at all. It only makes things worse.

So *learned* ways are what make the difference. So what? Learned ways can be unlearned. Identifying and unlearning your troublesome ways will free you to move toward your potential for self-actualization.

When it comes to really changing, one simple belief must dominate all others: "I can become the person I want to be; I am in charge of my life." Think about it. This belief is the basis for persistent motivation and the tool to avoid discouragement. Rather than feeling insecure about change, focus on the positive, delightful picture of you as you want to be—slim, vital, and in charge of your feelings and habits. When the challenge of personal growth wears you down, take a few minutes, relax, and re-create a successful, joyful image of yourself.

SOME TIME LEFT

How long has it been since you were really happy about your physical condition? It has probably been some time. It is a pretty toxic thing to be someone you really do not want to be. You know that the excess weight you carry is killing you and robbing you of your share of joy in life. You also know that you can lose that weight and be the sort of vital, happy, and attractive person who gets up in the morning with pride in self and who moves through the day with grace and dignity.

We probably all have an idea of just how long we will live. Another ten, twenty, thirty, or forty years for you? How are you going to live those years? Will you live them, really live them? Or will you just kill time for the next thirty years? Take some time right now to think about weight loss with respect to your whole life, not just the next three months. Where will you be a year from now, two years from now? Will you be ten pounds heavier, or will you turn things around and be the person you really want to be? You have the rest of your life ahead of you. Why not spend it in a way that brings joy and love and productivity?

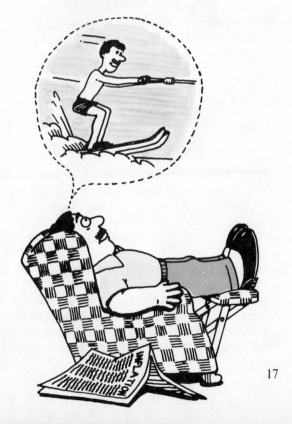

Take some time right now and relax. Sit back and create a vision of yourself. Make it as real as you can. Think about how you will look, how you will feel, and how clothes will look on you when you lose that weight.

Do not kill the possibilities by telling yourself that it cannot be done. Each moment you are a new and improved you. Just because you have not dieted successfully in the past does not mean you cannot do it now. You are learning and growing each moment, and you *can* do it!

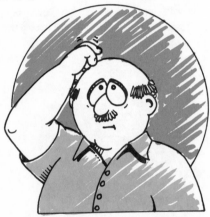

When driving a car, you have to look ahead. You have to look down the road some distance in order to steer properly. If you do not steer toward a point distant enough—if you try to steer by looking at a point too close to the car—you find that it is impossible to steer.

Keeping your motivation to lose weight is like steering a car. You have to focus upon the long-term success that will surely come rather than on the day-by-day learning process that is necessarily laced with some steps backward. If you lose sight of that long-term goal of success, you will become unnecessarily discouraged.

That discouragement is *always* a danger to be avoided. Keep your eye on the long-term goal and be patient. You will be successful.

THE MYTH OF A SINGLE CAUSE

The trouble with many diet writers is that they look at the problems of weight loss in only one way. They see only a one-dimensional problem, caused by one thing. Consequently they specify one treatment: suppress the appetite, reduce calorie intake, relieve the chemical imbalance, stabilize the blood sugar, or modify eating habits.

Being overweight involves not just one but all of the above problems. Yes, it is a problem of metabolism, because carrying excessive weight causes metabolism and body chemistry to change. Yes, it is a problem of nutrition, because fat is built up by excessive energy being stored, and to control weight the balance has to be reversed. Yes, it is a problem of limiting certain foods, because certain foods are addictive and actually cause hunger. Yes, it is a problem of exercising, because an effective energy level requires exercise. And because overweight people want to hide, to deny their bodies because they are embarrassed by being seen in public, it is most of all a psychological problem.

Because the needs and feelings and habits of overweight people played an important role in their becoming overweight, those elements must be changed to achieve a more effective life-style. But do not be discouraged. The fact that there are several causes gives us several effective starting points.

A COMPLEX AND EMOTIONAL THING

As a veteran dieter, you see the problem from a different angle than most diet writers. You know that weight control is a complex, emotional, highly per-

19

sonal experience, punctuated with times of loneliness, discouragement, and despair. You have tried all the magical keys to diet success, and you realize that it is much more difficult than diet writers seem to think.

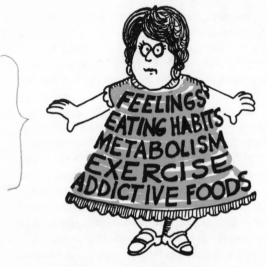

You also know that being overweight is not simply a case of increasing the chances of high blood pressure, heart disease, diabetes, varicose veins, and atherosclerosis. Being overweight is not just a condition that will close you out of better jobs and kill you years before you ought to die. It is all of these things, but it is more. Being overweight is a condition that robs you of the joy of accepting, respecting, and loving yourself. It separates you from others and robs you of the pleasure of living in a vital, healthy, and attractive body.

The drives and feelings you experience about yourself and food are a crucial part of the problem. Dealing with overweight, then, means learning some things about drives and feelings, and learning some things about yourself.

20

Things could be better. But try not to run to the refrigerator for a few hundred calories of security just because the problem is complex. There is another side to the story. With the help of several disciplines, the problems can be unraveled and solved. And you are up to it. You can even do it without living in an eternal state of self-deprivation.

YOU ALREADY HAVE MANY OF THE TOOLS

Think about it for a minute. You have had diet success at times. You have lost weight. Those periods of self-sacrifice have already shown that you do have the *will* to accomplish your goal. The times you lost weight were times of toughness and strength. Even when you put on weight, you still exercised restraint. You are not some kind of moral cripple, so get that idea out of your head right now. It only hinders your progress. You are a person who learned some habits that brought unhappiness and made you unhealthy. Tens of thousands of people have changed their habits. So will you.

Your desire to be the happy and healthy person you were meant to be will provide the motivation you will need. And with a certain amount of training, you will build the cheerful persistence needed to become slender and stay slender.

change feelings by changing thoughts

If being overweight is not a matter of simple chemistry or if it is not some kind of moral weakness, then what is it? Overweight is a complex phenomenon involving both the physical and the psychological sides of the personality. Behavioral habits and feelings lie at the core of the problem. The problem is that overeating, like other learned behavior, is strengthened by practice until it becomes an unconscious habit wrapped in layers of feeling that make it difficult to change.

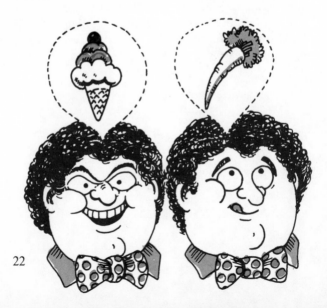

Once we begin to practice the overeating habit, it is strengthened by some powerful rewards. The relief from hunger, the pleasures of taste, and the short-term feeling of security that comes with a full stomach all reinforce the robot-like behaviors of eating.

But to say that eating behavior is at the core of the overweight problem is not to say that this is where the problem always begins or that it constitutes the whole problem. Overweight is not just a problem of habit, so to attack the habit without attacking some other important aspects of behavior is to make the mistake of "one cause." Several other aspects of the person are involved. Habits; the physical condition of being overweight; beliefs about self and about food and dieting; feelings of discouragement, loneliness, and even depression; and the tone of relationships with other people are all involved.

Look at the following circle:

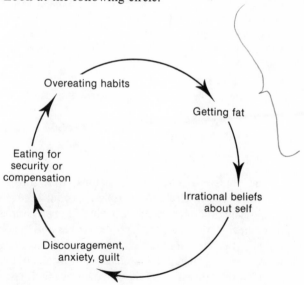

Does it look familiar? You can start anywhere in this circle and get into trouble. In the past, approaches to weight control have been single-minded. They attacked a single aspect of the circle. The idea seemed to be that if one problem in the circle were corrected, then the other problems would correct themselves. That was true in theory, but researchers are now recognizing that the more successful approaches attack the problem from several angles at the same time. One of the most successful approaches is taken by the Stanford Eating Disorders Clinic. In that clinic, patients are taught various aspects of nutrition, exercise, habits, and feelings. The successes are very gratifying and a new circle emerges:

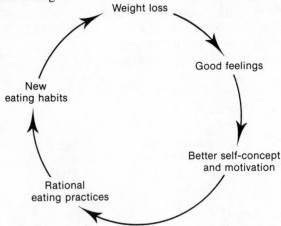

The goal is to change the vicious circle into the personal-growth circle. As people move into the personal-growth circle, some amazing things happen. They begin to love and accept themselves and, consequently, become more loved and accepted. They have more vitality, are happier, and have more control over their lives in other ways. They move toward their vision of a new self.

TRANSFORMING DISCOURAGEMENT, FEAR, GUILT, AND DEPRESSION

Cognitive therapy is an exciting new and powerful approach to dealing with unwanted, troubled, and driving feelings. As we have seen, feelings play a crucial role in the vicious circle. The questions are: Where do the feelings come from? How can I control them?

One of the early and still most popular proponents of cognitive therapy is Albert Ellis, who developed an approach to the repatterning of driving feelings called Rational Emotive Therapy.

Ellis describes Rational Emotive Therapy in a simple three-step model:

1. Unwanted feelings are the result of holding some irrational beliefs about self, the world, or other people. Such beliefs cause some experiences to result in troubled feelings. For example, many people maintain the irrational belief that they are not responsible for their overweight condition by repeating to themselves: "I'm not like other people; it's so easy for them" or "I just can't control myself." That irrational belief and kind of "self-talk" make for a limping self-image and lead to feelings of self-pity, frustration, and self-hate.

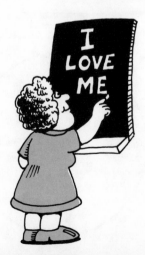

25

2. To change the feelings, the beliefs must be changed. That makes the whole problem much more manageable. Beliefs can be changed by changing the self-talk inside ourselves. Look at the following example:

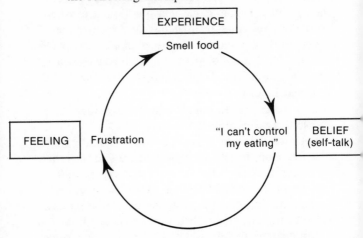

When you change the belief by changing the self-talk, the feelings automatically change. As you persist with new self-talk, the belief gradually changes and a new attitude emerges.

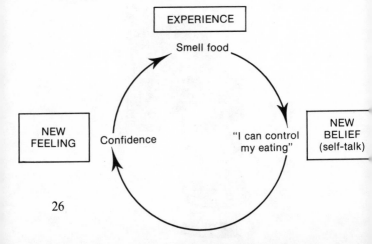

26

3. To improve one's emotional life, then, <u>one must</u> <u>attack the irrational beliefs by disputing them</u>. Once the attack has been successful, the person is free to establish sensible beliefs and appropriate behaviors. The unwanted feelings then go away.

It seems too simple to work, but Rational Emotive Therapy is a powerful approach to the problem of developing new patterns of feeling and rooting out deeply implanted unwanted feelings. It has been especially successful when used against depression—one of the most persistent mental-health problems and one of the key feelings in the vicious circle of overweight.

In the following chapters you will find a number of exercises to help you become aware of your unconscious and destructive self-talk. These will help you build a new and powerful vision of who you are. With intelligent and resolute work you will transform yourself, take charge of your feelings, and control your weight.

Please spend some time on the exercise following this chapter.

Discovering Your Self-Image

Self-image is based upon what we tell ourselves and the extent to which we believe our self-talk. It is useful to examine what we tell ourselves about who, what, and how we are. Answer the following questions by placing a YES or NO in the blank spaces. Your honest answers will help you identify what you believe about yourself and why you hold these beliefs.

1. If you have always been overweight do you:
   A. credit heredity for your body size? _____
   B. believe that you can control your body size? _____

2. Do you think of yourself as a "fatty," "tank," "hippopotamus," or the like? _____

3. Do others have affectionate yet unkind nicknames for you such as "chunky," "chubby," "tub," "blimp," or "lard"? _____

4. Did your parents believe that some people were born to be fat? _____

5. Did your parents tell you that you were going to be "just like your two-ton Aunt Lucy"? _____

6. Concerning willpower, do you think of yourself as:
   A. weak-willed? _____
   B. usually weak-willed? _____
   C. usually strong-willed? _____
   D. strong-willed? _____

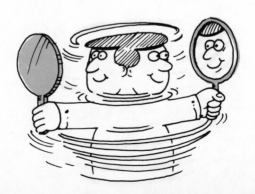

7. Do you feel that if you do not eat three good meals a day you will get sick?_____

8. Do you feel that if you are sick and have a loss of appetite you should force yourself to eat anyway?_____

9. Do you say to yourself that since grocery-store food is often refined and processed, you are not likely to get all the nutrients you need unless you eat large portions of everything?_____

10. Do you feel wasteful if you do not eat everything on your plate?_____

11. If there are leftovers after a meal, do you eat them because you do not want to "waste food"?_____

12. Do you eat rapidly?_____

13. Do you eat because it is time to eat, regardless of whether you are hungry or not? _____

14. After meals, do you usually feel stuffed? _____

15. Do you eat when others eat, whether you are hungry or not (for example, while watching TV or at social gatherings)? _____

16. Were you taught that unless you ate a good meal (cleaned your plate), you could not have dessert or a snack later? _____

17. Did your parents brag about what a good eater you were because you ate so much of everything? _____

Answers to these questions will help you understand both what you tell yourself about your fate, health, and willpower and where your learned eating patterns originated. The negative things you say to yourself are probably not true, and with a little practice you will be able to dispute them and replace them with positive self-talk. Negative self-talk erodes motivation, lowers self-esteem, and increases the likelihood of failure to

lose weight. Positive self-talk reverses
that and makes dieting easier and more enjoyable.
It also enhances self-image.

You are probably your own severest critic. Criticizing
yourself hurts, and it is usually not helpful in improving
attitudes, feelings, and behavior. It is more helpful to
talk good sense to yourself.

SOME FURTHER READING

Ellis, A., and Harper, R. A. *A Guide to Rational Living*. Hollywood, Calif.: Wilshire Book Co., 1968. The authors discuss the link between feelings and thoughts, ways to think ourselves out of emotional upsets, and how to accept reality, control our own destinies, become creative, and live rationally.

McMullin, R. E., and Casy, W. W. *Talk Sense to Yourself*. Denver: Jefferson County Mental Health Center, 1977. This book gives a basic outline for cognitive restructuring. Its aim is to help the reader quickly identify and overcome irrational thoughts with positive self-knowledge.

Maultsby, M. D., and Hendricks, A. *You and Your Emotions*. Lexington, Ky.: Univ. of Kentucky Medical Center, 1974. The authors provide cartoon illustrations of the basic emotional self-help principles and techniques used to help people clean up their "internal dialogues." The book offers pleasant insights into our unwanted emotions and shows us what we can do to change them.

build a positive self–image

As we saw in the last chapter, psychologists have established the relationship between how we think and how we feel and act. Who we think we are is an especially important aspect of the experiencing-thinking-feeling-behaving cycle. The thoughts you have about yourself—your competence, your social acceptability, and your sense of personal responsibility—influence how you interpret the things that happen to you and how you feel about and, consequently, respond to those things.

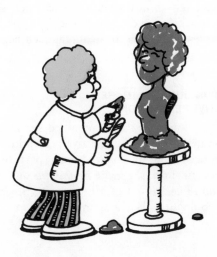

To see how this works, let us look at an example. Cynthia came to the authors' workshop discouraged and complaining that she could never lose weight. She had been overweight for several years, and she insisted that she did not have the strength or willpower to stick with a diet. She would diet for a couple of days, lose a pound, but then become discouraged and go on an eating binge.

As counselors talked with her, it became apparent to them that she thought of herself as weak-willed, unattractive, and unable to cope with her life. This, then, was the key to her feelings and behaviors. Her negative thoughts led to periods of extreme discouragement so that when dieting became uncomfortable, she would go on an eating binge—just as she believed she would. It was a self-fulfilling prophecy. She predicted the binge, and because she believed she would go on a binge, she did. Her belief led to the binge, and the binge reinforced the belief. A vicious circle.

Cynthia's perceptions of herself did not square with reality, however. She had two children, was a good mother, and enjoyed the friendship of several people who thought of her as friendly and competent. In reality Cynthia was not weak and unattractive but kind, hardworking, and caring. The question then was: What was she doing to maintain such negative thoughts about herself?

WE MAINTAIN OUR SELF-IMAGE
BY SELECTIVE PERCEPTION

One of the ways Cynthia maintained her negative beliefs about herself was by selective perception, that is, she noticed and internalized only part of her experiences. In short, she made *mountains* out of her failures and *molehills* out of her successes. She could diet for two or three days at a time and do very well, showing admirable self-control and willpower. But somehow she failed to internalize and relish her successes. She did not use her successes to build a positive self-image, but instead used her failures to feed a negative self-image. As soon as she overate on her diet she would blame herself, calling herself weak-willed and careless. Her feelings of discouragement followed, and she was off on that old vicious circle again.

UNRELENTING STANDARDS

Many people maintain negative self-images and negative feelings by setting unrelenting standards for their own behavior. In the language of Transactional Analysis, they have a severe Parent. No matter how good, competent, kind, strong-willed, or loving these people are, they are never good enough for themselves. Their own unrelenting standards set them up for failure because they can never quite live up to them. This means that no matter how good they are, such people only see failure in themselves and have no realistic way of building a positive self-image.

Overweight people do this by setting absurdly unrealistic goals. "I'm going to lose four pounds a week for ten weeks!" That is an unrealistic goal for most people—the kind that sets dieters up for failure, because as soon as they miss the mark for one week, they feel that they *are* failures. So the cycle of discouragement and eating returns again. One small disappointment wipes out days or weeks of success.

CHALLENGE YOUR PERCEPTIONS AND STANDARDS

As soon as Cynthia was taught to recognize her selective perception and her unrealistic personal standards, she could challenge them and start building a more positive and more realistic self-image. Subsequently her feelings and behaviors changed. (The

33

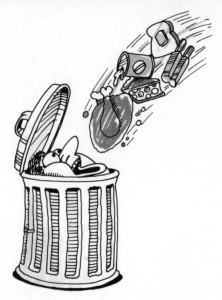

Molehill Journal found on pages 42–43 will help you
examine your own perceptions and standards.)

To recap it then, your beliefs, your feelings, and your
behaviors are uniquely and predictably tied into "who
you think you are." You can find out who you are in
relation to weight loss by answering some questions.

* How much willpower do I have?
* How much of my weight problem stems from my
  parents?
* Why do many other people have no problem
  staying trim?
* How do I look?
* What do others think about my being fat?

WILLPOWER IS A CRUCIAL PART OF SELF-IMAGE

What did you say to: "How much willpower do I
have?" If you have selective perception and rigid
personal standards, you will feel weak-willed. Your
answer may have sounded like this: "My willpower is
only good occasionally. It's good when I'm full, and it's
poor when I'm hungry." Can you recognize any

destructive self-talk here? There is nothing constructive in thinking of yourself as weak-willed. As a matter of fact, thinking about yourself that way just gives you an excuse to *not* lose weight.

It goes further than that, however. If you tell yourself that you are weak-willed, you will feel helpless and this helplessness will trigger eating. Again the old vicious circle emerges. Do not put yourself down with labels like "weak-willed." Just start noting your successes and feel good about them.

BE HERE, NOW

Are or were your parents fat? How about Aunt Lucy? Did your family give you a model of poor eating habits? Did they make you clean your plate "because of all the starving people in the world"? Did they urge you to eat when you were sick, tired, or unhappy about something—subtly suggesting that the panacea for all ills was to E-A-T? These are all formative aspects of your life and probably influenced your answer to: "How much of my weight problem stems from my parents?"

But simply telling yourself that your overweight condition is your parents' fault is spending today looking backward. It does not help much because it gives you the impossible burden of changing the past before you can change the present. And as far as we know, the past cannot be changed.

The present, however, is a different matter. You can formulate plans and direct your actions toward learning new habits in the present. And that is what it takes to lose weight.

Live in the here and now. Do not blame your past. Yes, it is true that your problem behaviors started then. But let the past die. You *can* learn to control your eating as of now.

DO NOT BLAME YOUR FAT ON OTHER PEOPLE

"Why do other people have no problem staying trim?" Perhaps they are just lucky. Perhaps they have an extremely rapid metabolic rate. Whatever the reason, dismiss the question. It just leads to a cop-out.

If you envy slim people and assume that their life is easier, you are probably right—not because of luck or metabolism, but simply because they learned a better set of habits and beliefs about food and dieting. You can learn those habits and beliefs yourself.

Do not make the mistake of assuming that you are an "unfortunate." Being "unfortunate" tempts you to feel sorry for yourself. That breeds self-pity and leads to self-talk about what a "pitiful" person you are. That vicious circle again!

YOUR BODY IMAGE IS PART OF YOUR SELF-IMAGE

Does your fat detract from your appearance? Did you answer the question "How do I look?" with some derogatory statement? If you tell yourself you are ugly, you are saying you are a person no one likes. Most people are repelled by ugliness, any kind of ugliness. If you have ugly clothes, you grow to despise your wardrobe. If you say you are ugly, you will grow to despise yourself. Once you hate yourself, how will you ever be able to do anything good for yourself? Saying you are ugly and hating yourself for it is loaded with self-destructiveness.

How did you answer "What do others think about my being fat?" If you assume that they dislike your fatness or hold you in low esteem because of it, you will feel rotten. You could get around the feeling by saying that others are cruel, or you could agree with their judgment. Then both you and the others would be holding you in low esteem.

36

Either of these ways is likely to make you unhappy. Do not focus attention upon the negative aspects of your relationships with others. Rather, take comfort in the fact that there are many people just like you and that both you and they have friends.

YOU CAN CHANGE THAT SELF-IMAGE

The most important question to ask yourself is: "Who do I think I am?" If you think you are poorly motivated, you will feel poorly motivated. If you think you are weak-willed, you will feel helpless. If you say you cannot overcome temptation, you will feel weak. If you blame your past, you will feel victimized and incapable of acting responsibly. If you say you are unfortunate, you will pity yourself and feel pitiful. If you think you are ugly, you will build self-hate and be unwilling to lift a finger to help yourself. If you say that others are cruel or that they do not like you, you will feel rejected and unhappy.

If some of this self-talk fits you, you can bet that you will have some pretty negative feelings. The person you think you are, at least at this moment, might be described something like this. "I am a poorly motivated, helpless, weak-willed, irresponsible, pitiful, angry, unhappy, rejected person." That is such a destructive self-image that you may want to eat yourself into an early grave just to get away from yourself.

If your self-talk is based upon irrational beliefs, then it will explode into destructive feelings and become an obstacle for you. You do not have to be destructive and build unwanted obstacles for yourself. You control your own thinking. When you recognize that, you can begin to choose thoughts which are based on reality— thoughts that will enhance you and lower the barrier between you and becoming "who you want to be."

37

To further explore your self-image, please do the following exercises.

Personal History

This worksheet is designed to heighten your awareness of factors that may have contributed to your present body image.

1. At what age did you begin to think of yourself as overweight?

_____

2. What brought your attention to your overweight condition?
(Put a check mark after conditions that apply.)

A. Seeing myself in a mirror or photograph. _____ ✓

B. Parental comments. _____

C. Spouse's comments. _____

D. Sibling comments. _____

E. Peer comments. _____

F. Having to buy "fat" clothing. _____ ✓

G. Wearing a swimsuit in public. _____ ✓

H. Physical-education classes. _____ ✓

I. Inability to be as physically active as others. _____

J. A doctor talking to me about dieting. _____ ✓

K. Weight gain during pregnancy. _____ ✓

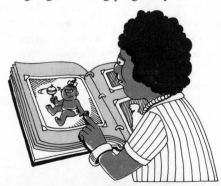

3. Weight at different ages in your life (Check appropriate boxes.)

AGE	OVERWEIGHT	WEIGHT OK	BODY IMAGE Good	OK	Poor
0 – 5					
5 –10					
10–15					
15–20					
20–25					
25–30					
30–35					
35–40					
40–45					
45–50					
50–55					
55–60					
60–65					
65 plus					

4. History of dieting.

A. At what age did you first diet? _____
B. Other attempts at dieting. (Check appropriate boxes.)

AGE at DIET	SUCCESSFUL	UNSUCCESSFUL	BODY IMAGE Good	OK	Poor
25	✓			✓	
30	✓		✓		
35		✓			✓

5. What attitudes do you have about other people's body size? (Check appropriate boxes.)

	Disapprove	Do Not Care	Like It
Spouse			✓
Mother		✓	
Father	✓		
Brothers	✓	✓	✓ ✓
Sisters			✓
Friends	✓	✓ ✓	✓ ✓
Employer			
Co-workers			

Are these attitudes important in maintaining your own body image? _____

6. What attitudes do you believe others have about your body size? (Check appropriate boxes.)

	Disapprove	Do Not Care	Like It
Spouse	✓		
Mother		✓	
Father	✓		
Brothers	✓ ✓	✓ ✓ ✓	
Sisters	✓		
Friends	✓ ✓	✓ ✓ ✓	
Employer			
Co-workers			

Do the attitudes of these people shape your own feelings about your body image? _____

Looking back over this questionnaire, does it suggest to you why you hold the body image you now have?
_____

An Awareness Exercise To See How I Interpret Things To Maintain My Self-Image

In the boxes below, briefly outline either the negative or positive self-talk you honestly believe you indulge in.

	NEGATIVE SELF-TALK	POSITIVE SELF-TALK
Think of a specific time when you have shown toughness (such as finishing an especially difficult assignment), when you sacrificed for someone, or when you worked hours to please someone.		
Think of a time when you wanted to do something that you had not done before.		
Think of a time when someone gave you a special kind of compliment.	*Nice Lunch at My Home*	
Think of the times when you visualize yourself as successful at dieting.		
Think of a specific time when you have been successful at dieting.	*32 1986 - Canada*	

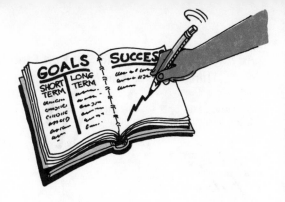

The Molehill Journal

You have seen that people maintain their self-image by selective perception, that is, they make mountains out of their failures and molehills out of their successes. Cognitive therapists have had very good success in helping people change their self-images and their feelings by having them keep a journal of successes. They ask individuals to record, in objective fashion, the successes they experience each day. In this way, people will begin to stop making molehills out of their successes and start giving themselves credit for them. An easy but effective strategy.

Here is what the authors would like you to do. Get a spiral notebook or some other handy album. Each day spend some time with your journal. Write about three kinds of things.

First, write to yourself about who you would like to become. Record your thoughts about your general and long-term goals in this section.

Second, set down specific, short-term objectives for yourself. These short-term objectives should be steps toward your long-term goals. Make them realistic and manageable.

Third, keep a record of your successes in achieving your objectives. Write to yourself about how you feel about your successes. Reverse that destructive self-talk and practice being the optimistic person you really are.

You may want to pattern your journal after the sample on the following page.

Molehill Journal

(sample page)

1. My long-term goals (who I would like to become) are:

Wear comfortable clothes

jeans

Belted fashions

petite - Size 14

2. My specific, short-term objectives for today are:

Lose 10 pds

3. My successes and accomplishments today are:

Cereal

Salad - Soup

salad.

make friends
with your feelings

There is probably not an overweight person in the world who was not told as a child to eat everything on his or her plate "because there are children starving all over the world." That saying lives on in us. When we try to leave the table without cleaning our plates, we feel just a little bit guilty. We are haunted by old sayings that have shaped our habits and our bodies.

To some extent our feelings are tied to those old sayings. To change our feelings about ourselves and about food and dieting, we must necessarily bring those old sayings into our consciousness and put them to rest. Many of those old sayings were based upon conditions that existed in the past. Those of us who are middle-aged or older were brought up in hard times when good food was expensive. People genuinely feared malnutrition and undernutrition. It was very important at that time for children to be impressed with the idea that they ought not waste food. It was both an economic and social imperative.

Times have changed, however, and most of us can afford good food. In fact, most of us buy much more food than we really need. Our task is rather to reduce our food intake. Those old moralistic sayings simply get in the way of our progress toward becoming happier and healthier persons.

DR. JEKYLL AND MR. HYDE AT THE REFRIGERATOR

Probably everyone who has struggled with weight control has experienced an internal conflict or a feeling of tension about being on a diet. You feel as if you are two personalities: a Dr. Jekyll who knows and understands the problems of weight control and who has a commitment to losing weight, and a Mr. Hyde who wants to eat you into an early grave. As you stand in front of the refrigerator, Mr. Hyde urges you to eat anything and everything in sight, no matter what the taste, no matter what the consequences. Just eat. At the very same time, Dr. Jekyll thinks rationally and coolly about your desire—your very real desire—to lose weight. Dr. Jekyll tries to restrain Hyde, but sometimes Hyde has too much energy and is too strong. So the hungry monster wins and you wind up going on a binge. Even though the thoughtful, rational part of you sometimes wins and you avoid the binge, you always live with the fear that Mr. Hyde will go on a rampage at any time.

Transactional Analysis (TA) is a theory of social psychology that helps us understand and deal with the Jekyll and Hyde that lurk in us. It shows us how it happens that we have the desire to eat more than is

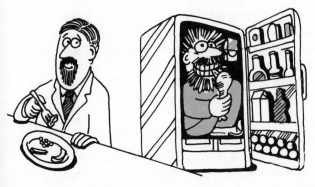

necessary for maintaining weight and experiencing maximum vitality. More importantly, TA shows us how to turn off the old, unhealthy parts of our personality so that we can live more rational and more joyful lives.

TA therapists have had excellent results working with people who have the Jekyll-and-Hyde eating syndrome. They show us that different parts of us grow out of how we learn. Old, destructive patterns based upon ideas our parents gave us, or fears and feelings we had as helpless and dependent children, replay from deep inside us. These old patterns complicate the task of really taking charge of our own lives. The goal, then, is to become conscious of those old patterns of feelings, beliefs, and behaviors—to sort through them and turn off the troublesome ones.

For example, one woman whom TA therapists worked with used to "sneak eat" at night when her husband was working and the children were in bed. She was asked in class to consciously identify her feelings when she was "sneak eating." She said that she had a feeling of rebellion while she ate. Gradually the therapists found out that the woman's mother used to hide food from her when she was a little girl. When she found the hidden food, she would eat it to spite, or punish, her mother.

Her "sneak eating" was a replay of old feelings and old behaviors. After a short discussion, she realized that the old feelings and old behaviors were not punishing anybody but herself. The situation had changed, but the old pattern of rebellion continued. She sorted out that pattern and finally rejected it.

THERE IS A PARENT IN US

Psychologist Eric Berne has shown that the human personality is a complex thing made up of three rela-

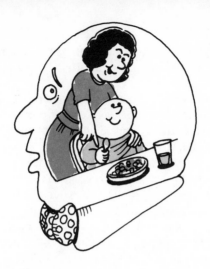

tively distinct parts called "ego states." When conducting group therapy, Berne noticed that the people in his group had three voices: one like a child, another like a parent, and the third much like the adult voice used in normal conversation. Upon further investigation he saw that along with different voices, each person had a specific set of beliefs and behaviors that went with each voice.

As he thought about what he observed, he began to form a theory based upon the idea that the brain records all our experiences. The different voices and behaviors we manifest are "playbacks" of things we have heard from our parents and others. Our feelings are often playbacks of feelings we experienced as a child. This theory explained a lot of things about why we go on binges and why we feel guilty.

The Parent ego state is the recording of the ways our parents spoke and acted toward us when we were children. We have internalized the Parent (our own parents) within ourselves, and at times we find ourselves speaking their slogans and in their tone of voice. When we find ourselves mouthing the old slogan, "Eat

47

everything on your plate—there are children starving all over the world," we are functioning in the Parent ego state.

The Parent in us also tells us *when* we ought to eat. You might remember, as a child, your mother looking at you worriedly and saying, "You're tired, you need something to eat." This recording can set up a basic pattern for you. Whenever you feel fatigued, you respond to that feeling by going to the refrigerator and eating whatever you can get your hands on.

The Parent in us, then, is a very important part of our personality and something that needs to be analyzed thoroughly. At the end of this chapter you will find a worksheet to help you get in touch with some of the recordings in your Parent. Those recordings are often forgotten, but they just as often are what maintain our habits. The point of the worksheet is to bring those recordings into your consciousness so that you can sort them out, keeping the ones that are still appropriate and discarding those that are archaic and destructive.

THERE IS A HUNGRY CHILD IN US

During the first five years of our life, we had very close contact with someone who "parented" us. He or she set our basic patterns of behavior in relation to food. Each time we were told what to do or what not to do, we had a "feeling" response to the statement. When we were told that we were naughty for not eating our spinach, the Child part of us responded with some feeling—probably a feeling of shame, maybe a feeling of rebellion. So the Child ego state is a series of recorded feelings that are linked with the things that are said in our internal Parent. When the Parent in us says, "Eat everything on your plate, there are children starving all over the world," the Child in us responds by

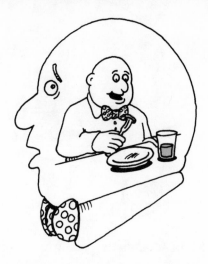

eating everything on the plate and feeling guilty if anything is left.

The Child in us is also very important because it is that part of our personality that represents the physical part of us. The Child in us is very sensuous and almost always hungry. The Child in us sometimes fears starvation. This can be a rather grim and deep-seated belief causing us to respond to the prospect of skipping a meal or not getting enough food with feelings of fear and foreboding.

The Child in us is also the part of us that "sneak eats." Many dieters have a habit of stopping at a grocery store and picking up a "snack" of a pound or so of salted cashews and eating them on the way home. It is impossible to keep that up and lose weight.

The Child in us is the seat of many of the feelings that are troublesome when we go on a diet. Getting to know our Child, then, is a very important part of moving toward our vision. One of the worksheets at the end of this chapter asks you to think about some of the things that happened when you were a child that may determine some of your eating habits now.

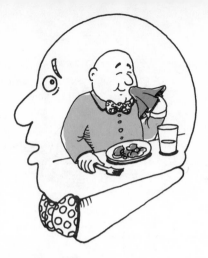

THERE IS AN ADULT IN US

The Adult is the part of our personality that starts to develop as we learn language. The Adult is the least emotional part of us and is the most logical or rational part of us. When we start to go on a diet, the Adult sets the goals and lays out the menus.

Both the Parent and the Child are simply recordings that are played back in our heads. The Adult, on the other hand, functions more like a computer. The Adult weighs evidence and makes judgments in a more complex way than either the Parent or the Child. This makes the Adult an effective tool for intervening in the behaviors of the Parent and the Child.

THE ADULT CAN EDIT PARENT AND CHILD TAPES

When the Parent recording "Eat everything on your plate, there are children starving all over the world" is played, the Adult ego state can intervene and show that leaving something on your plate does not cause other children to starve at all. As a matter of fact, there is no relationship between the food you leave on your plate and another person's nutrition. The Parent in us would lead us to become a kind of human garbage can. Our Parent would have us eat for the sake of an abstract moral principle, "Don't waste food." The Adult shows us that our health and happiness are more dependent upon dieting than saving imaginary children in some far-off place.

One of the important functions of the Adult ego state is, therefore, to intervene in the recordings of both the Parent and the Child and to dispute them on logical grounds. This process is what Albert Ellis calls "disputing irrational beliefs." We will talk more about that in Chapter 7.

Now take some time to become more conscious of your Parent and Child by doing the exercises that follow.

Discovering Your Parent Tapes

Answer YES or NO.

1. Did your parents lay down rules about eating everything on your plate?

2. Did your parents tell you that wasting food was wrong or sinful?

3. Did your parents encourage you to eat by telling you all the good things food will do for you?

4. Did your parents emphasize the scarcity of food?

5. When you were ill, did your parents give you special food treats?

6. Did your parents often eat between meals?

7. Did your mother or father take particular pleasure in eating desserts?

8. Did your parents reward your special behavior with sweets?

51

Revealing Your Hungry Child

Answer YES or NO.

1. Do you ever experience fear when you skip a meal? Can you trace that feeling to your childhood?

2. Do you "sneak eat" when you are alone? Can you determine when you learned to do this? (Specify.)

3. When you feel tired or lonely, do you automatically go for food?

4. When you feel anxious, do you run to the refrigerator?

5. What other feelings trigger your eating? (Specify.)

6. Does food give you a sense of security?

7. Do you feel that you have a hungry Child in you?

SOME FURTHER READING

James, M., and Jongeward, D. *Born to Win*. Reading, Mass.: Addison-Wesley, 1971. Very good treatment and application of Transactional Analysis for personal self-understanding. Especially useful for many overweight individuals is the section on "The Drama of Life Scripts."

Phillips, P., and Cordell, F. *Am I OK?* Niles, Ill.: Argus Communications, 1975. The authors focus on people's OK-ness by facilitating the readers' awareness of each person's inherent potential. They help the reader understand how to move in a positive direction by looking at how to use time, relate to others, and contribute to the well-being of self and others.

CHAPTER 5

Age 12 -
Mom 16½ - I woul I
(Some day -
Sat. nite Candy as a Kid.

develop
a healthy life script

We have already talked about how important your self-image is in the struggle against overweight. Both Eric Berne and Claude Steiner have shed some light on how the self-image is formed. They argued that early in life, in the Child ego state, most people make a potent decision about their life course. They decide who they are and who they are going to become. That decision becomes an important part of their self-image and, in some instances, a powerful driving force in their lives.

Berne and Steiner called this unconscious life plan a "life script," because the behavior of the person is played out to achieve some dramatic end. For instance, a young boy who is called stupid (in a number of subtle and sarcastic ways) by his parents because he is having trouble in school might make the decision that he is *in fact* stupid. He then plays out that life script throughout his life by paying special attention to the mistakes and errors he makes rather than to the intelligent and creative things he achieves. In fact, he might play certain psychological games like "Stupid" in order to reinforce his life script. His behavior and his internal dialogue would also reflect and reinforce his decision that he is stupid.

"Stupid" is a tragic script because it destroys people and robs them of the joy of intelligent and creative action. It is self-destructive. Suicide, alcoholism, and

53

insanity are intense forms of tragic, self-destructive life scripts.

For fat people, the life script is based on the dos and don'ts and labels laid down by their parents. Such things as "Clean up your plate" and "You are just like Aunt Lucy, she was doomed to be fat" have a powerful effect on the young mind. That is why it is important for you to get in touch with your own Parent ego state. In your Adult, sort through the statements and discard the destructive ones.

If you experience a deep-seated feeling of fatalism, if you feel that fate demands that you be fat, you may be struggling with a fat life script. But do not run off to the refrigerator for compensation. Life scripts can be changed. And you can change yours.

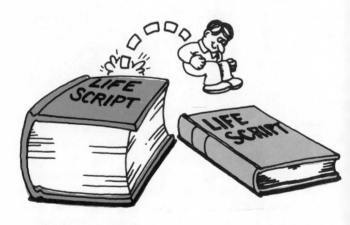

PULLING CLEAR OF A FAT LIFE SCRIPT

The first thing you can do to pull clear of a fat life script is to learn to love your body. After all, it is your home—the only one you will ever have. You only hate your body because your Child thought that self-hate had the benefits of no responsibility and it got pity from others. You know better now, so start changing.

The fat person faces a paradox. In order to change your life, you must be motivated. You must want to be different than you presently are. On the other hand, if you base the desire to change on self-hate you are caught in a trap. The self-hate triggers bad feelings which you compensate for by eating and eating and eating. But the paradox is not real. Healthy change starts with self-love. Motivation comes with the realization that self-fulfillment is possible for all people, even fatties. In order to change, then, you must want to change but still love yourself the way you are.

Steiner says that people with fat life scripts must learn to say "no" and to express anger. He argues that fat people feel that they have to "swallow everything." Because of this, anger builds up and such people tranquilize themselves with food. We will deal with some ways to say "no" in Part 3.

The fat person must also get in touch with his or her body. This means learning to "listen" to feelings and sensations and to trust them. Eat when you are hungry. Learn to rest instead of eating when you are tired. Learn to talk to someone instead of eating when you are lonely.

Most of all, give up self-hate. This means turning around the toxic self-talk. Start telling yourself the truth: You are a beautiful, precious, onetime occurrence in a pretty big universe.

In order to change your life script, begin to examine your Parent tapes and your Child tapes by completing the following worksheet.

A Life-Script Exercise

This exercise is designed to help you remember things that might have led you to build a fat life script. Write your answers in the space provided.

1. Do you ever remember deciding that you had to be a fatty? *No*

2. Do you have the feeling that you were "born to be fat"? *N1*

3. Do you find it hard to say no to people in authority?
Y

4. Do you remember things your parents said that led you to believe you were doomed to be fat?
Y

5. What nicknames did people call you? What did the names mean to you?
–

6. What do you like the least about yourself?
waist-line

7. Do you ever feel that something might be wrong with you?
Y

8. Does it seem to you that sometimes you go out of your way to find something to feel badly about?
Y

9. What in your life do you feel worst about?
weight, Tommy – David did. Steve   No kids

10. What do you like most about yourself?
energy, talented, ability to do things

Can you now identify things that led up to a decision that your life was destined to be plagued by fat?

56

let go of
unwanted feelings

**FEELINGS THAT MOTIVATE SOME PEOPLE,
TRAP OTHERS**

Somewhere along the line every overweight person has experienced large doses of discouragement and the feeling of being trapped in an unhealthy and unappealing body.

These unwanted feelings usually lead directly away from a weight-loss program. So *feelings* about being overweight are often a real barrier to the weight loss we so dearly desire. The feelings themselves are part of the vicious circle:

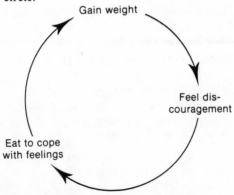

Gain weight

Feel dis-
couragement

Eat to cope
with feelings

'Round and 'round we go. And rounder and rounder we get!

To most of us it is not surprising news that feelings are a problem. Problems can be solved by sorting out our feelings about ourselves, about food, and about eating and by changing our patterns of feeling so we can get out of that vicious circle. Happily enough, there are some powerful and well-substantiated techniques for doing just that. The following discussion is an introduction to those techniques.

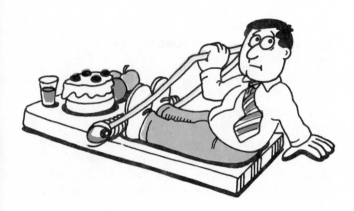

GETTING OUT OF THE TRAP

The goals of this and the next chapter are to show three important things:

1. Our feelings and behaviors—especially our feelings of discouragement and our urges to go on binges—are directly connected to some irrational Child or Parent beliefs about ourselves, about food, and about eating, and those feelings are triggered by certain routine events.
2. Those irrational beliefs of ours were learned early in life, and they continue largely because we hold onto them.

3. Having chosen to discontinue those destructive beliefs, we *can* change them by conscious, unrelenting, and vigorous effort.

The part about changing is the most important point in the whole scheme. The part about beliefs and feelings must be understood before we can get down to the task of rebuilding our patterns of feeling.

In order to get there, we again refer to the work of Albert Ellis.

FEELINGS ARE TIED TO SELF-TALK

Albert Ellis and other cognitive therapists have shown us how feelings are connected to our self-talk, that is, the things we believe. In this model, events do not lead directly to feelings. Seeing a cherry pie does not make you feel hungry directly, but the hungry feeling comes from some beliefs through which you interpret the sight of the pie. Specifically, you might believe that the pie will bring you pleasure. That belief is *not* true, because eating it will bring more excess weight and bad feelings.

It works something like this:

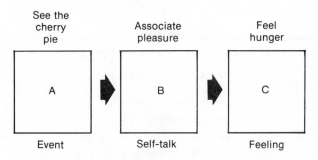

The feeling (C) is usually followed by some behavior. We have a feeling and then we act upon it. In order to show this, we can add another box to the model presented by Ellis:

59

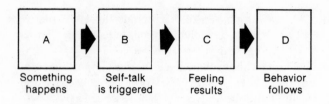

A	B	C	D
Something happens	Self-talk is triggered	Feeling results	Behavior follows

Let us see how this works for the habitually over-weight person.

Something happens:
The clock shows 12:00 noon.

Self-talk or beliefs:

1. "I *need* to eat three full meals a day or I will get sick."

2. "When I'm hungry I can't control my eating, and because of that I'm not an OK person."

Feeling: Anxiety and defeat

Resulting Behavior:
Stuffing

Example 1

In Example 1, the noon whistle (activating experience) does not directly cause the anxiety or the stuffing. Whistles by themselves have no power to cause feelings (anxiety) or behavior (stuffing). The feeling and the behavior result from the irrational beliefs held by the overweight person. Your slender co-worker does not get anxious or begin stuffing when the whistle blows. Why not? Because he or she has different beliefs. Your beliefs are what cause the problem, and they can be changed.

The second example focuses on a different belief and a different situation.

You overeat on your diet by 200 calories.

1. "I *know* I never can stay on a diet. I always set goals and am too weak to meet them."

2. "If I go off the diet even a little, I have ruined that day, so I can only start over tomorrow."

Discouragement

Eating binge

Example 2

In this example, it seems as if the eating of 200 extra calories caused the feeling of discouragement which led to an eating binge. However, it is the belief that "I'm weak" or "I've ruined the day" that is the cause of feeling discouraged. Eating 200 calories, when isolated as an activating event, can be seen as having no power to cause any emotion. It is what you say to yourself that causes the feeling. The 200 calories are insignificant, while your self-talk is highly significant. An irrational belief such as "200 calories makes a great difference" is simply destructive thinking. Developing rational beliefs helps build constructive self-talk, good feelings, and appropriate behavior.

The first step in building more positive feelings is to bring your beliefs into your consciousness. This is done by asking yourself what your self-talk is. The following exercise is designed to help you get in touch with your self-talk.

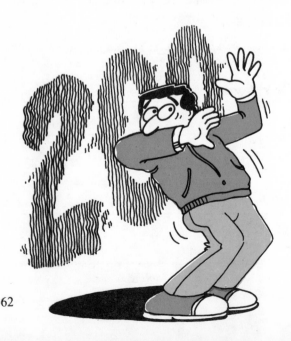

Dealing with Feelings

The goal of this worksheet is to help you uncover irrational childhood beliefs related to yourself, to eating, and to dieting. Write your responses in the space provided.

1. About self-control and eating, I tell myself:

too Hard to Control — all or none

2. About the sacrifices of dieting, I tell myself:

Doesn't seem to be worth it

3. About why I am overweight, I tell myself:

its temporary — Later I'll Lose Weight

4. About physical health and eating, I tell myself:

feel better when I eat healthy

5. About calories and weight control, I tell myself:

Needs to be too strict

6. About why other people I know are not overweight, I tell myself:

Don't have as many problems.
Can't control it when I travel

7. About skipping a meal, I tell myself:

will get a head ache

8. About getting started on a diet, I tell myself:

Next week, when I stay in Fla
for a long period of time

9. When I am in the middle of an eating binge, I tell myself:

tastes good

10. About being the person I really want to be, I tell myself:

soon I'm going to lose weight

SOME FURTHER READING

Greenwald, J. *Be the Person You Were Meant to Be.* New York: Dell, 1973. The author distinguishes between "nourishing" and "toxic" living and helps the reader develop antidotes to types of self-induced toxic situations, such as loneliness.

Powell, J. *Fully Human, Fully Alive.* Niles, Ill.: Argus Communications, 1976. A very readable book about how our "vision" shapes our lives. The author talks about common misconceptions and the sources that create our perceptions of ourselves, others, and the world around us. A key point throughout the book is that improving our self-talk leads to being "fully human, fully alive."

dispute
destructive self-talk

We may want to let go of beliefs that lead to destructive feelings and behaviors, but somehow we find it is not so simple. The Parent and the Child hold onto the irrational beliefs and reinforce them in an internal dialogue between the three parts of us—the Parent, the Child, and the Adult. These beliefs are also reinforced in the ways we structure our time and relate to others.

No overweight person has escaped the experience of one part of the self crying out for a snack and, at the same time, another part of the self responding, "If you want to lose weight, you must forego such things." So the internal dialogue, or self-talk, goes.

As we have seen, some self-talk helps us hold onto old and unhealthy ways of believing and behaving. Unhealthy self-talk related to overeating we will call "fat self-talk." We will contrast this fat self-talk with "healthy self-talk." Let us look at the following examples:

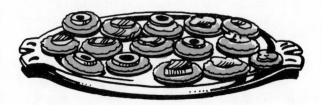

```
┌─────────────────────────────────────────────┐
│             Irrational Childhood Belief       │
│         "I know that I cannot stay on a diet." │
└─────────────────────────────────────────────┘
```

Examples of fat self-talk that hold onto the belief	Examples of healthy self-talk that help us change

"I'm not like other people."

"Other people are really quite similar to me. They control their weight, and so can I."

"All I have to do is look at a piece of cake and I put on weight."

"I'm a strong person. My weight loss is not dependent upon other people understanding me."

"Nobody really knows how hard it is to stay on a diet."

"I can stay on a diet, and I will."

As mentioned in Chapter 4, this process of replacing fat self-talk with healthy self-talk is what Ellis calls "disputing irrational beliefs."

Self-talk is so much a part of us that we often have trouble putting our finger on it at first. Some people recognize their self-talk right away, while others must work to recognize it.

FAT CAN BE A RACKET

A general principle of psychology is that behavior patterns are strengthened when they are rewarded or reinforced. Knowing this, one wonders what possible benefit people derive from a pattern of toxic self-talk. The answer comes from the work of Eric Berne.

Ironically some people do derive benefit from their irrational beliefs and self-talk. For instance, if you hold onto the belief that you will *never* be able to lose weight, you derive two benefits: (1) you avoid responsibility; after all, if you really cannot lose weight, you have no responsibility to try and (2) you get the benefit of sitting around companionably with others and playing "Poor me" and "Ain't it awful?"

Deriving benefit from some destructive habit or belief is what Eric Berne called "a racket." Check yourself out: Are you using your fat to avoid responsibility or to get sympathy from others? If you are, dispute those benefits. They are short-term benefits, and in the long run they block your progress toward self-actualization.

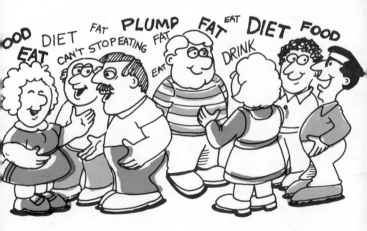

THE WAYS WE STRUCTURE TIME ARE IMPORTANT

Eric Berne argued that people have two basic motivating psychological hungers: We hunger for recognition, and we hunger for stimulation. Both of these hungers are satisfied by positive encounters with other human beings called "strokes." Since we need strokes so badly, we structure our time to insure a good supply of strokes.

For overweight people and dieters, this often means getting together with other overweight people and discussing the problems and difficulties of dieting. Such discussions can take either a toxic bent (where they reinforce negative beliefs and negative self-talk) or a positive, productive bent (where discussions revolve around goal planning, productive approaches, and success in a positive, optimistic tone). The results of those choices are obvious. If we choose to be negative and pessimistic, the encounter will feed the vicious circle. If we choose to be positive and optimistic, we will not only get the strokes we need but also help ourselves into the personal-growth circle.

The worksheet at the end of this chapter is designed to help you bring to your consciousness the Child and Parent beliefs about yourself, about food, and about eating that lead to unwanted feelings.

A word of caution: It is sometimes difficult to be honest with yourself, especially about things like being overweight. Your feelings are strong and confused; it takes a while to sort them out. The overweight person is apt to want to blame someone, but it does no good to blame anyone—least of all yourself. As a young child you probably learned to solve problems by eating. You can change that now by being persistent. Blaming yourself will only create a lot of fat. Remember, persistence pays off.

Dealing with Feelings

The goal of this worksheet is to help you uncover unrealistic Child and Parent beliefs and to consider some other, more effective, beliefs. Take a few minutes to "listen" to yourself as you write your response to each question. Then repeat the replacement belief to yourself.

1. Do you tell yourself that you will **never** have the self-control needed to solve the problem of weight control? What do you say to yourself?

+ Would be a life time of needed control

Try telling yourself that <u>you have exercised self-control many times before and that you will strengthen your self-control by practice and self-analysis.</u>

2. Do you tell yourself that dieting is not worth the sacrifice? What do you say to yourself about the sacrifices of dieting?

Last 20 yrs dieting hasn't worked

Try telling yourself that you **can** enjoy diet food. In fact, you will enjoy it more because you will learn to eat more slowly and savor your food. As a result you will feel much better, have more vitality, and be more attractive.

3. Do you tell yourself that you were born to be fat just as Aunt Lucy was? Do you tell yourself that <u>your fat is inherited</u>? What do you say to yourself about your condition?

Dad was fat — Brothers + sisters   *His*

			weren't
Ruby	Eddie		Orville
Alice	Hank	Edith	Rollie
Esther	(7)	Elluena	Donald
Lillie		(8)	Marvin
			Russell

69

Try telling yourself that if fat is an inheritance, you want to be cut out of the will. Tell yourself that you have learned some inappropriate eating habits that have led you to become overweight and that you can and will learn healthier eating habits.

4. Do you tell yourself that dieting will make you overtired or sick? What do you say to yourself about physical health and eating?

will get a head ache

Try telling yourself the truth: that improved diet will help you become stronger and more vital in every aspect of your life.

5. Do you tell yourself that you cannot keep track of those calories and that they make no difference anyway? What do you say to yourself about calories and weight control?

eating out its impossible to tell

Try telling yourself that you can reduce the calories in your diet—and do so easily—by avoiding sugar and fats and limiting carbohydrates.

6. Do you tell yourself that other people are different—that they can eat all they want and still stay slim? What do you say to yourself about why other people are not overweight?

More important to them
Don't travel as much

they

Try telling yourself that slim people have achieved an excellent energy balance, just as you are going to do.

7. Do you tell yourself that you will starve if you miss a meal? What do you say to yourself about missing a meal?

_____

_____

_____

Try telling yourself that you already have lots of meals stored away for a rainy day—and today it's raining.

8. Do you tell yourself that today is already ruined, so you will have to start tomorrow? What do you say to yourself about getting started on a diet?

when I have the time & energy
to do it

_____

Try telling yourself that you can start eating more appropriately anytime. The sooner the better.

9. Do you tell yourself that you are a crazed demon when you are on a binge? What do you say to yourself when you are in the middle of a binge?

I won't do this tomorrow

_____

Try telling yourself that you can stop anytime, that stopping is good, and that you will be better off the sooner you stop.

10. Do you tell yourself that you never will be able to be the person you want to be? What do you say to yourself about being the person you really want to be?

Slim can't be done —
easier to change my attitude
just accept the weight as is

71

Try telling yourself that you are getting better and better—that you are good and tough, and that you **will** be who you want to be.

Now, go back through these ten items and ask yourself the following questions:
1. Am I using this particular belief to avoid being responsible for my life or in order to get pity?
2. Am I using this particular belief to cement my togetherness with my fat friends?

Return to this exercise once in a while, and remind yourself to practice more positive self-talk.

Structuring My Time with Other People

Many people who struggle with weight control fall into bad habits in their conversations with other people. Two of the things people "pastime" about are "Ain't it awful we can't lose weight?" and "Ain't it awful that we can't control ourselves no matter how hard we try?" The purpose of this worksheet is to help you assess the ways you structure your time with others.

1. List six people you spend time with talking about food, diets, and weight control.

A._____   D._____

B._____   E._____

C._____   F._____

2. How much of your conversation is self-defeating talk about how "I will never make it" or "how hard I have tried and still failed"?

_____

_____

_____

3. What steps can you take to stop playing "Ain't it awful?" and begin engaging in conversations and pastimes that involve positive self-talk?

_____

_____

_____

walk
bridge
tennis

PART TWO

BEHAVIOR MODIFICATION AND WEIGHT CONTROL

A thirty-year review of the literature of the traditional treatment of obesity shows a dismal picture: No more than twenty-five percent of patients treated lost as much as twenty pounds.

Behavior modification is an approach to learning new habits. When linked with cognitive therapy, behavior modification enables more than ninety percent of dieters to be successful.

Good! There must be something to it.

Keep a journal

get to know your robot

Have you ever caught yourself standing at the refrigerator half an hour after a good meal picking through the leftovers? Overweight people commonly eat when they are not hungry. The question is, Why? There is a "robot" in each of us. It is part of us. Our Robot is the thing that stands in front of the refrigerator and eats cold hot dogs when we are not even hungry. Our Robot also responds to feelings of anger, frustration, loneliness, or fatigue by running to the refrigerator and eating the leftover apple pie. Sometimes our Robot whispers in our ear, "You're tired; you need something to eat" or "You don't feel well; have something to eat and you will feel better."

Each of us has a Robot in us. The Robot has a powerful effect on the way a human being learns and behaves. Even though the Robot is troublesome, we need it. It relieves us of a tremendous burden when we carry out routine tasks like driving a car, tying our shoes, buttoning a button, or recognizing acquaintances on the street. Our Robot responds immediately and automatically to the cues and directions we give it. If we had no Robot, our minds would be filled with a thousand details and we would have little time to be fully human.

WE PROGRAM OUR ROBOT

Do you remember when you started learning to drive? At first, you had to think about every single operation: press down the clutch, put the car in neutral, insert the key in the ignition, and so forth. As you backed out of the driveway and started down the street, you had to consciously concentrate on each move. When you started to go too far to the right, you had to correct it consciously. This conscious effort went on for quite some time. After a while, however, you found yourself driving down the street without even thinking about it. This happens when the Robot takes over.

By concentrating on the task of driving, our Robot has been programmed. Sooner or later it conveniently takes over for us. This is fortunate, because after the Robot takes over, we can get into our car and say, "Let's go down to the shopping mall." Next thing we know, we are there. We just punch in the directions and our Robot drives us there automatically. It leaves us free to think about other things, to sing, to talk, to listen to the radio while we are driving.

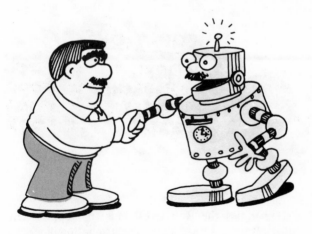

ROBOT HABITS ARE TRIGGERED BY CUES

The Robot functions in many aspects of our lives by responding to various cues in our environment. Sometimes the cues are visual impressions from our environment. We see a red light and put our foot on the brake. Sometimes the cues are conscious directions like getting into the car and saying, "Let's go downtown." This is the Robot at its best, responding to the directions we consciously intend to give.

The Robot of the overweight person often responds to the sight of food by eating, even when not hungry. The image may not even be of real food. A picture, a commercial on TV, a wooden pear—anything triggers eating in the fat Robot.

For the overweight, the time of day is often a cue to eating. The Robot responds to the noon whistle and the dinner bell even when the person is not hungry. Perhaps it is not so bad to have a Robot that is triggered three times a day. But what about four, five, or twelve times a day?

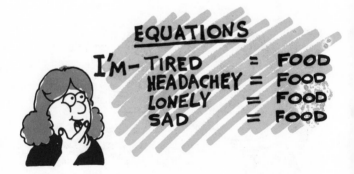

Sometimes the Robot responds to inappropriate internal cues, such as fatigue, a headache, loneliness, or sadness. The Robot recognizes the feeling as a cue to eat, which subsequently leads the overweight person further into the unwanted feeling.

The Robot links eating with certain places. Obviously the kitchen table and the dining-room table are places that present visual and olfactory cues. The problem is that overweight people link many other places with the reinforcers associated with eating: the car, the motion-picture theater, the couch in front of the TV, the bedroom, the bathtub—anywhere and everywhere.

Finally, the Robot links certain events with the pleasure of eating. Often such pastimes as visiting with friends or watching TV triggers automatic eating. When this is the case, the Robot must be reprogrammed.

Behavior modification is based on a simple principle of psychology. We learn to do things more often and more intensely when we are rewarded for doing them; and we are less likely to learn things when we are not rewarded or are punished for doing them. Reinforcements are of various kinds. Sometimes reinforcements are social, such as a pat on the head. Sometimes reinforcements are subtle, such as the fulfillment of some need or a pleasureable experience. Sometimes reinforcements are planned, conscious experiences; sometimes they are less conscious. Sometimes we rely on others to reinforce our behaviors. Sometimes we reinforce our own behaviors.

Reinforcement gives us the primary tool for reprogramming our Robot's inappropriate eating behaviors. "Reprogramming" in this sense means trying to reduce certain kinds of behaviors or substitute other kinds of behaviors. Since we are conscious of our own goals, we can set up programs to reinforce the Robot in new ways and consequently change its behaviors.

79

The first step in reprogramming the Robot is to become aware of its patterns of behavior and consciously recognize the events, people, times, and feelings that trigger inappropriate eating. This recognition gives us the basic information needed to start working on reprogramming the Robot. For instance, many of us respond to feelings of fatigue by eating. The blood sugar goes down, we feel a little bit tired, and we immediately go to the refrigerator for a snack to increase the blood sugar. When we have a little snack, the blood sugar goes up and the tiredness is alleviated somewhat. The alleviation of that condition reinforces the habit of eating to deal with fatigue. But there are other ways to deal with fatigue: rest, sleep, or exercise. There are a number of things that can be done to raise the blood sugar. To repeat, then, the first step is to recognize what triggers the eating behavior and what reinforces it.

The second step is to eliminate the reinforcement that has shaped our inappropriate behavior. The third step is to substitute a new habit and reinforce that habit with a consciously chosen reinforcer—some reward.

COLLECT DATA ON YOUR ROBOT

You will need to collect data in order to help you see more clearly the habits of your Robot. You will be asked to keep a ten-day record of the things you eat, how much you eat, the times when you eat, the places where you eat, how you feel and what other activities you are engaged in while eating. It is absolutely crucial that you keep accurate records. Measure your food. Record every snack or bit of food you eat. Try to determine what feelings trigger eating.

As we have seen in other chapters, we deny or distort painful experiences. It is not easy to accept the fact that we are in charge of our lives. Many times we hide things from ourselves and actually lie to ourselves. We try to escape from the fact that we are overweight. We exaggerate how hard we try to diet, but we forget about the snacks we sneak. Collecting data in an honest and straightforward way is the vital first step in the process of changing your Robot.

Self-acceptance is the fundamental starting point in change. As long as we do not accept ourselves, we cannot fully recognize our patterns of behavior. If we fail to recognize our patterns of behavior, we cannot change them. So it is important that you record anything and everything you eat. Be absolutely sure of the amounts you eat, without overestimating or underestimating. The very fact that you become conscious of how much you are eating will help you reprogram your Robot. So, collecting baseline data is important in two ways. First, it raises our consciousness of the amount of time and energy we put into eating. Second, it provides the basic material for the analysis needed to start the change process. In the following pages you will find a journal. This journal runs for ten days. There are six columns for each day.

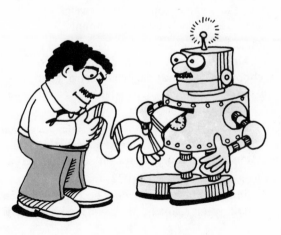

Column 1 is to be used to record *what* you ate and drank. Record everything in detail. Make sure that when you have three cheese crackers at two o'clock in the afternoon, those go down as having been eaten. Some people tend to forget what they drink because they do not define drinks as food. Liquids often count up to hundreds of calories during the day. One woman who said she never ate breakfast added: "Of course, I drink two large glasses of orange juice every day." Somehow she did not define orange juice as food. Yet two large glasses of orange juice contain as many calories as a medium-sized breakfast.

Column 2 is to be used to record *how much* was eaten. Overweight people often underestimate the quantities of food eaten. Sometimes they underestimate because they have taken too many helpings and so they forget the amount. Sometimes, however, they may not really be conscious of just how large a medium-sized apple is, for instance. When you eat one of those softball-sized apples, be sure that you record it as such. Some diet groups demand that people actually weigh their food on a small postal scale. These scales can be obtained in most department stores. If you are unaware of how much you are eating, weigh your food and learn to accurately estimate amounts.

Column 3 is to be used to record the places *where* you eat. Do you eat standing over the sink, in your car, in the shopping mall, in an easy chair in front of the TV, at the dining-room or kitchen table? Record accurately where you are each time you eat.

Column 4 is to be used to record the times *when* you eat. Two kinds of data are important here. One is the actual time when you eat; the other is the actual amount of time you spend eating.

Column 5 is to be used to record how you *felt* when you ate. Did you feel lonely, tired, sad, anxious, angry, sorry for yourself? Just make a note of how you felt each time you ate. The data will make you conscious of the feelings that trigger eating.

Column 6 is to be used to record *other activities* that are tied to eating. Were you watching TV? Were you chatting with friends? Were you alone in the house? Other activities are often systematically linked to eating.

Carry your journal with you for ten days and keep accurate records of your eating habits. Baseline data about your "normal" eating patterns must be collected before you go on a diet. Use the time you are collecting data to begin other exercises in the book. Begin working on the feeling patterns that trigger inappropriate eating. Start building your motivation and working on your self-image. A little over a week from today you will feel better about yourself and be ready to start a diet—an effective and successful program of weight control.

Day 1

1 What Did You Eat/Drink?	2 How Much?	3 Place?	4 Eating Times Begin　　End	5 How Did You Feel?	6 Other Activities

Day 2

1 What Did You Eat/Drink?	2 How Much?	3 Place?	4 Eating Times Begin End	5 How Did You Feel?	6 Other Activities

Day 3

1	2	3	4		5	6
What Did You Eat/ Drink?	How Much?	Place?	Eating Times Begin End		How Did You Feel?	Other Activities

Day 4

1 What Did You Eat/Drink?	2 How Much?	3 Place?	4 Eating Times Begin End	5 How Did You Feel?	6 Other Activities

Day 5

1 What Did You Eat/ Drink?	2 How Much?	3 Place?	4 Eating Times Begin End	5 How Did You Feel?	6 Other Activities

Day 6

1 What Did You Eat/ Drink?	2 How Much?	3 Place?	4 Eating Times Begin End	5 How Did You Feel?	6 Other Activities

Day 7

1 What Did You Eat/ Drink?	2 How Much?	3 Place?	4 Eating Times Begin End	5 How Did You Feel?	6 Other Activities

Day 8

1	2	3	4		5	6
What Did You Eat/ Drink?	How Much?	Place?	Eating Times Begin	End	How Did You Feel?	Other Activities

Day 9

1 What Did You Eat/Drink?	2 How Much?	3 Place?	4 Eating Times Begin End	5 How Did You Feel?	6 Other Activities

Day 10

1 What Did You Eat/Drink?	2 How Much?	3 Place?	4 Eating Times Begin End	5 How Did You Feel?	6 Other Activities

SOME FURTHER READING

Fanburg, W., and Snyder, B. *How to Be a Winner at the Weight Loss Game.* New York: Ballantine, 1975. A behavior-modification book set up to help the reader accurately record food consumption and analyze what occurs concurrently with eating. Helpful ideas are offered about learning to eat more slowly, avoiding distractions that lead to overeating, and becoming aware of "influences" upon eating, such as feelings, places, and people.

Robbins, J., and Fisher, D. *How to Make and Break Habits.* New York: Dell, 1976. The authors describe behavior modification and help the reader apply it to breaking habits, including the habit of overeating.

Stuart, R., and Davis, B. *Slim Chance in a Fat World.* Condensed ed. Champaign, Ill.: Research Press, 1972. A book on behavioral control of obesity. The authors draw heavily from behavior modification to help the reader design a good weight-control program. They cover nutrition, exercise, and behavioral control of eating habits.

psychological tools and creative options

In previous chapters we have talked about how to change patterns of feelings in a purely conscious way. That material was based on Transactional Analysis and Rational Emotive Therapy. The tools described in this chapter are those used primarily by behavior managers.

REINFORCEMENT

Behavioral theory hypothesizes that people learn to do things habitually that they are often rewarded for doing. For instance, a child who gets a piece of candy to reinforce "good" behavior will learn to be good in order to get the reward.

We all use positive reinforcement to shape our own behavior. Dieters, for example, reward themselves when they stay on a diet or when they behave in some desired way. The reward links good feelings with the new behavior. As we make that association, we tend to behave in that new way more often.

Some reinforcements are used to discourage certain habits. One famous weight-loss clinic uses a timed electric spoon to help people slow down their eating. When dieters put spoons into their mouths too rapidly, they get a mild electric shock. People then begin to connect a mild distress with eating rapidly. Waiting

eat slowly

long enough between bites does not produce a shock. This negative reinforcement teaches the Robot to eat slowly.

Reinforcement, then, becomes a powerful tool in shaping our own behavior. Or, to put it another way, reinforcement is a powerful tool in reprogramming our Robot.

CHANGING HABITS

The habit of eating too rapidly, mentioned above, has a couple of unfortunate consequences. First, people eat much more than they are consciously aware of eating and, second, they overfill their stomachs before the sensation of hunger goes away. Consequently, they eat far more food than they need in order to satisfy the physical sensation of hunger.

Even without an electric spoon, you can devise ways to eat more slowly. Learn to set your fork down between bites, chewing the food thoroughly. Consciously focus on eating slowly the same way you focused on steering a car when you were new at driving. Eventually the habit will change. Rather than stuffing and eating very rapidly, your Robot will become programmed to eat more slowly.

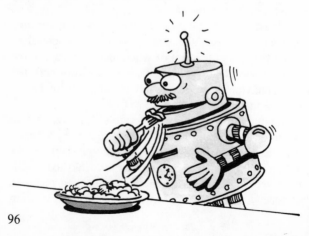

Often when people practice a new skill they feel that they are doing something alien to themselves. It does not feel good at first. This is a natural consequence of doing something you are unused to. Do not let that feeling deter you from practice, however. Anyone who has learned to drive a car, play an instrument, or use a typewriter knows that it does not take long before the skill grows by leaps and bounds.

VISUALIZATION AND SYSTEMATIC DESENSITIZATION

As you become aware of your eating behavior, you will find that there are certain times when it is especially difficult to curb your eating. For instance, the sight of a smorgasbord laden down with food triggers Robot stuffing.

Such behavior can be changed by utilizing "visualization experiences." Relax and imagine yourself going to a party where there will be a smorgasbord. Try to create a very realistic and vivid visualization of the physical situation. What is the room like? What does the food look like? Now try to examine your feelings during the party. What are your feelings as you enter the room? What are your feelings as you approach the smorgasbord and pick up a plate? Do you feel the impulse to pile the food on? Dispute that impulse, and imagine yourself taking moderate and appropriate amounts of food. Practice doing this. It takes only a few moments, but it will help you restrain your Robot "stuffer."

DESENSITIZATION IN VIVO

Visualization is fantasy. Reality is when you are actually *at* the party. Learning to control your feelings in a real situation is what psychologists call "desensitization in vivo."

97

Once you have built some confidence and set some goals in relaxed visualization, it is time to face the world. That means you must actually go to a smorgasbord party and try out your new-found confidence. It is important in a field test to maintain your concentration and avoid distractions. You must anticipate as many distractions as you can and develop a plan for dealing with them. If you fail to, your Robot will take over and run amok over the groaning board.

You must anticipate seeing your friends with heaping plates. You must anticipate that many of them will be "food pushers." They will say, "Ah, come on, just once. It won't hurt you." Anticipate such things in your visualization and think of specific things to say to people who invite you to overindulge in food "just this once."

SELF-CONTRACTING

Self-contracting is a way of systematically reinforcing yourself in order to change behavior. It means setting goals for ourselves, watching our behavior carefully, and applying positive or negative reinforcements as needed.

Self-contracting is an important tool because it helps us become acutely aware of our behavior and consequently helps us "move out of the Robot." But more than that, it provides a continuous positive reinforcement for shaping new behaviors.

Because self-contracting makes us aware of reinforcers, it also helps eliminate those things that reinforce our old unwanted eating behaviors. For instance, when we eat while watching TV, the pleasure of watching TV reinforces the eating behavior. Once we know about reinforcements, we can move to eliminate those things that reinforce old eating patterns.

The following worksheet is an example of a behavior contract.

Self-Contract for Eliminating Behavior
Remember:

1. Make your goals simple and operational, that is, things that can be observed. For example, "I will not eat at coffee breaks at the office."

2. Make your rewards things that will please you, such as some time to yourself, going to a movie, or buying something you have wanted for a long time.

The behavior I want to eliminate is the following:

Eat only at Counter or Dining Table - Sitting down

Each time I catch my Robot behaving in an unwanted way, I will score 1 point against myself. If I have no more than 2 points during the week, I will reward myself by doing what I have contracted for, which is:_____
I will then move on to a new behavior contract.

If I have more than 2 points, I will start over and get **no** reward.

ALTERNATIVES AND OPTIONS

Another way to stop our Robot's bad behavior is to develop alternatives and options to the destructive responses we make to cues. For example, when the clock strikes noon, one might go for a walk or read a book instead of sitting down to a big lunch.

When we create alternatives and options, we free ourselves from the immediate and automatic responses to cues in our environment. This, in fact, gives us a high degree of freedom. And it is much healthier to eat only when hungry rather than in response to cues.

DEEP RELAXATION

As we have seen in previous chapters, many people respond to anxiety and other internal sensations by eating. Deep relaxation is a technique used by behavior therapists to help people get in touch with their physical sensations and reduce anxiety. It helps us sort out our various sensations and attach new responses to them.

Deep relaxation can be used many times during the day. It is an especially helpful tool to use prior to mealtime to slow ourselves down and help us concentrate on our goal of personal growth and weight loss.

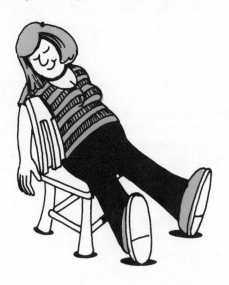

Prior to relaxing, you should gather together some positive thoughts that will enhance motivation, self-concept, and healthy living. When you have chosen the thoughts, enter the deep state of relaxation. Take from ten to twenty minutes to get relaxed. At the point of total relaxation, you are in a highly suggestible state sometimes referred to as an "autohypnotic state." It is during this state that you repeat those positive thoughts.

RELAXATION EXERCISES

As you approach relaxation, make yourself comfortable. Close your eyes and focus your attention on your hands. Clench your fists tightly and hold the tension. Now relax. Let all the tension drain out of your hands.

Now tense your forearms and hold the tension. Now relax. Notice the difference between the tensing and relaxing. Tense your biceps. Then relax them. Just relax for a moment. Now tighten your neck muscles. Push your head back against the chair or bed and notice the tension in your neck. Now relax your neck.

Use the same procedure moving from head to toe. For example, tense your forehead by frowning, your eyes by closing them tightly, your jaws by biting down. After tensing each area for five seconds or so, take five to ten seconds to let the tension drain away and the relaxation flow in. Tense and relax the muscles already mentioned as well as these:

shoulders	hips
upper back	buttocks
lower back	thighs
chest	calves
stomach	feet and toes

Once you have gone through these major muscle groups, both tensing and relaxing them, return to any which are not relaxed and tense and relax them again. As your whole body becomes relaxed, you have heightened your state of suggestibility and are ready to whisper those positive thoughts to yourself. The suggestions will be more potent because of your relaxed, suggestible condition.

101

After learning the art of deep muscle relaxation (usually three to six practice sessions), you may be able to eliminate the tensing and simply direct your consciousness to each of the muscle groups and instruct them to relax. This works just as well and takes less time, although most of us learn the process best by beginning with the tensing.

USING POSITIVE SELF-STATEMENTS

Examples of helpful positive thoughts during relaxation are:

"Instead of eating I'm resting, and that is healthful."

"Staying on this diet will trim me down."

"By eating less, I'm getting closer to wearing more attractive clothing."

"My appearance will improve as I continue my diet."

"I'll be adding years to my life by losing weight."

"Weight loss is easy; it's simply a matter of putting less into my mouth."

"When I stop relaxing, I will not be hungry."

Choose your own motivational and positive statements. Once you have a few in mind, relax all the muscle groups in your body and quietly say each thought to yourself four times. Then go back to relaxing. Relax for a minute, keeping thoughts at a minimum and focusing on the comfort of being relaxed. After a minute of relaxation, choose another thought and repeat it four times, slowly. Continue this procedure until you have whispered all the thoughts you have chosen. At the end, relax again for one minute and then quietly say to yourself, "I'll count backward from 4 to 1; when I reach 1, I'll open my eyes and feel refreshed and rested."

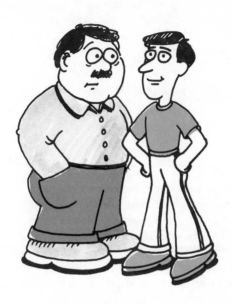

You should practice this at least once every day and continue to choose thoughts that you feel will help you most.

LEARN FROM MODELS

Most overweight people can make a very long list of individuals they wish they could be like. Psychologists call this "idea modeling." Modeling is simply becoming aware of and imitating the behavior of people we respect and wish we could be like.

In our society, people who maintain an ideal weight have often developed strategies or tricks to maintain proper eating habits. We have much to learn from them. As has been pointed out, overweight people tend to sit around with other overweight people, reinforcing the old fat ideas with toxic time structuring. Modeling means restructuring our time with people who have healthy eating habits. Talk with them, spend time with them, and learn from them.

PRACTICE THOUGHT STOPPING

When you learned to drive a car, you found that your Robot quickly took over. This happened simply and automatically because you practiced all of the skills needed for driving. Practice is another important tool in building new behaviors.

As you know from experience, one event often leads to a thought about food, and that thought leads to the impulse to eat. For example, the smell of popcorn in a theater, the aroma of bakery goods, the sight of food at a picnic, or even an ad in the newspaper first triggers the thought of eating and then the deed. Even though it often does not seem so, we do control our thoughts. To effectively control eating, we must learn to stop thoughts about eating.

Psychologists use a technique called "thought stopping." When you become aware of thoughts about food creeping into your consciousness, stop them with either a thought of something very unappetizing, or think of some event, plan, or person who has great importance to you. Some people get excellent results from thinking about what eating and overweight do to them.

Each of us can conjure up some thought-stopping image. It may be something that has actually happened to us or something we have imagined. Think of some noxious smell, some disgusting image, or some event that turned your attention away from food.

The following are some examples of thought stoppers that people in the authors' workshops have used to divert attention from eating. One young man thought about eating a worm, a fat old night crawler. Another person thought of the fat that was building up around his heart each time he ate a caloric snack. When troubled with thoughts of some delicious morsel, one woman imagined herself as a rusty old garbage can. In a more positive vein, one person envisioned her new body—how she would look as she lost her excess fat.

It takes only a small amount of creativity to vividly imagine something that is incompatible with eating. You may find one thought stopper that works forever, or you may have to continually create new ones. The point is to learn to stop your troublesome thoughts about food before they become action. When you learn to stop those thoughts, the environmental cues will lose their compelling power over you.

CREATIVE RESPONSES

Overweight people are often in a rut. Their responses are linked with certain cues in an automatic sequence. Creative options are simply new responses to old cues. Instead of letting fatigue automatically trigger eating,

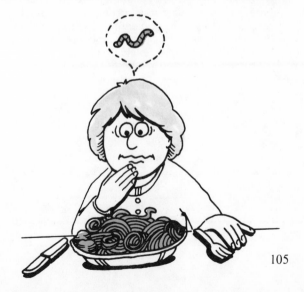

the dieter who consciously uses creative options takes a nap, does deep muscle relaxation, or takes a walk. Instead of allowing loneliness to automatically trigger a binge, the lonely dieter consciously replaces that response by calling a friend, reading a book, or going shopping. The person who eats when anxious must learn to cope with the anxiety by using such creative responses as meditation, quiet time, or exercise.

The task for the dieter is to develop alternatives and options to be used in place of old eating responses.

The next chapters focus on several aspects of behavior modification and are designed to take you through the major steps of a modification program. Please work through the following exercise before going on.

Creative Options

List as many activities as you can that you **like** to do and that are **not** linked with eating. Doing this exercise will bring you both an expanded awareness of activities you enjoy and a clearer appreciation of those that are least likely to involve eating. This information will be useful to you as you continue your program of modification. Here are some examples of creative options: jogging, knitting, bicycle riding.

_____	_____
_____	_____
_____	_____
_____	_____
_____	_____
_____	_____
_____	_____
_____	_____

_____   _____
_____   _____
_____   _____
_____   _____
_____   _____
_____   _____
_____   _____
_____   _____
_____   _____
_____   _____
_____   _____
_____   _____
_____   _____
_____   _____
_____   _____
_____   _____
_____   _____
_____   _____

SOME FURTHER READING

Benson, H. *The Relaxation Response.* New York;
   Avon, 1976. The author describes how to relax and
   lists the healthful benefits that accompany learning
   how to rid ourselves of tension and stress.

put exercise into your program

Imagine yourself walking on a magnificent beach. Water flows over your feet and the sun bathes your skin in warmth-giving waves. You have feelings of vigor and warmth and security. Imagine looking out across the bright blue water. The sun plays on the tips of the waves, blending the blue into shimmering bits of silver and gold. What a pleasant experience! Our bodies are potentially the source of an immense amount of pleasure. And each of us has a tremendous potential to increase that pleasure.

A rational approach to physical movement can help you become more aware of your environment through improved physical condition and an increased awareness of your surroundings. Increased movement can develop a greater sense of vitality and strength, more sensitivity to feelings, and a heightened awareness of the present moment. It can improve the cardiovascular system and forestall the aging process. No matter how young or old we are, we can develop our bodies so that we no longer struggle for breath, but instead have a sense of endurance and power.

Physical education has often promoted a rigorous, militaristic philosophy that better health can come *only* through sweat and pain. Most people who are overweight find this approach unappealing and threatening. They see themselves sweating down the street in their underwear with their fat bouncing up and down. They imagine their legs being chafed raw. They see themselves coming home with sweat pouring down inside their clothing and waking up feeling sore and uncomfortable. It does not have to be that way. Physical exercise can be pleasant and beautiful—like our walk along the beach.

START WITH WHAT YOU CAN DO

Many overweight people, then, are frightened by the prospect of an exercise program that causes them to suffer pain, agony, and a sore body. They especially retreat from the visibility of exercising in public. And because of this grim image, they do not even entertain the possibility of exercise. They deny it. In fact, some people try to psychologically deny their body in many different ways.

Some psychologists believe that obesity is motivated at the unconscious level by a desire to destroy the body.

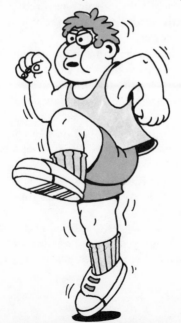

What is being proposed here is a love affair with your body. Learn to love yourself and your body. And in so doing, do the things that strengthen your body. Heighten your awareness in a positive and sensuous relationship with your environment.

GET STARTED BY INCREASING YOUR MOVEMENT

How do you get started? It is all quite simple. Do what you *can* do. Anything is better than nothing. Most people can walk. Start there.

One weight-loss group suggested some possibilities for improving movement. The following is just a "laundry list" that the participants proposed.

- At lunchtime, take a ten-minute walk before or after you eat.
- When you have a few minutes, take a walk through a park and watch the children playing.
- When you go shopping, park an extra block away from the shopping area and walk.
- Get up early in the morning, get dressed, and take a short walk around the yard of your house or apartment building.
- In the winter, savor cold air on your face and watch the sun rise as you take a short walk.
- Never miss a sunset.
- In the evening, take a short walk outside instead of snacking.
- Use the stairs instead of an elevator. Start by walking up one flight, then take the elevator on the second floor.
- Stand when you would normally sit.
- Take a break from work and go for a short walk each hour.

The individual suggestions do not amount to much exercise in themselves. But using a number of them will increase your daily exercise by a large percentage. This

110

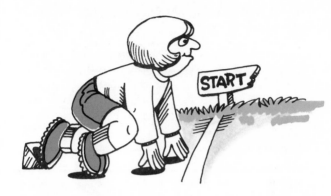

will help you tone your muscles and keep you away from temptation.

BE CONSCIOUS OF PHYSICAL MOVEMENT

Become more conscious of your physical movement, and move about more in your environment. Do what you can do easily, conveniently, and enjoyably. Do *not* involve yourself in an unrealistic exercise program. Avoid leading yourself to failure by setting unrealistic goals. Do not make yourself feel like a martyr by winding up with sore muscles or worse, but rather set a course toward involving yourself much more thoroughly in physical activity over the long run. Whatever your present condition, you should be moving about considerably more within a year. If you are young and not excessively overweight, you should be running or doing more vigorous exercise. Older or more obese people should progress more slowly.

A worksheet is provided to help you analyze your daily activities and set some realistic goals for yourself. Put a check mark or a "Yes" in the appropriate boxes to indicate the activities you normally indulge in at particular times of day. Total the number of times you did the activity. Please do this exercise as soon as possible.

Analyzing My Exercise Day

Type of Activity

	Lying Down	Sitting	Standing	Walking	Hard Labor	Playing or Running
6:00						
7:00						
8:00						
9:00						
10:00						
11:00						
12:00						
1:00						
2:00						
3:00						
4:00						
5:00						
6:00						
7:00						
8:00						
9:00						
10:00						
11:00						
12:00						
Totals						

I would like to increase my activity by doing _____

_____

My reward will be_____

_____

SOME FURTHER READING

Cooper, K. *The New Aerobics.* New York: Bantam, 1970. A book on how to begin a scientific exercise program, how much exercise is enough, and what benefits can be derived from numerous types of physical activity.

Leonard, Jon N.; Hofer, J. L.; and Pritikin, N. *Live Longer Now.* New York: Grosset & Dunlap, 1974. This book has excellent chapters on the relationships of diet to degenerative diseases. It shows how to develop an exercise program and introduces the concept of "roving."

Morehouse, Laurence E. *Total Fitness in 30 Minutes a Week.* New York: Pocket Books, 1976. An excellent treatment of the problems of building an exercise program by the man who devised the exercise program for NASA.

roving is an excellent alternative

There is much more beauty in the world than most of us ever realize. One way of getting in touch with that beauty is to walk. Many of us are not fortunate enough to live close to a beach or near the mountains where the scenery is awe-inspiring, but there is real beauty in our environment nonetheless. Part of learning to be the person you want to be is getting in touch with that beauty and at the same time learning to move about more in your environment. This can be accomplished through "roving."

Roving is simply covering ground. It means walking, jogging, running, or any combination of these. Indeed, one of the best approaches to exercise is simply walking.

At first you may be able to walk only a short distance. If you are greatly overweight, you may find that walking a block causes perspiration and shortness of breath. People in better physical condition can walk farther or even run a bit. The objective is to cover as much distance as you comfortably can.

Short walks increase our vitality by strengthening our muscles and building lung capacity. If we walk regularly, even for short distances, what was once a difficult walk becomes a pleasure. As the pounds melt away, you will find that walking becomes much easier and much more pleasant. This is especially true after six weeks.

Roving is an excellent tool in the personal-growth circle. It helps us avoid excess eating; it helps us feel better and actually speeds up weight loss.

Start with a physical examination by a doctor. After that initial examination, the best method for determining what exercise you can do is to "listen" to your body. Listening to your body means being aware of the signs of strain and fatigue. Excessively rapid heart rate, slow recovery of breath, and general exhaustion are signs that you need to slow down. You will know when you have reached the right level of exercise when you feel refreshed, revitalized, and energized by the walk or run.

If you are very obese and in poor physical condition, take heart. After a half-block walk, your lungs will be filled with fresh air, and that feels good. A half block now does not mean that you will always be limited to that distance. Your body will improve steadily because of exercise. As your body builds strength and endurance, you can increase the exercise.

Roving allows you to listen to your body and walk the distance that energizes you rather than depletes your energy. Eventually you may be roving four or five miles a day in addition to your regular activities which could involve another four or five miles of walking as you clean house, walk to your office, or go shopping. The authors of the book, *Live Longer Now*, suggest that you work up to ten miles a day to reverse the effects of degenerative diseases.

You can probably already walk a half block or more. Envision yourself a year from now, two years from now, on your program. Sit back, relax, and visualize yourself after you have attained your weight-loss goal and have developed new vitality. See yourself as slim and attractive. Imagine yourself being involved in bowling or playing tennis or taking long walks in a way that you never dreamed you could. Free yourself. Visualize your success.

You have the potential to enjoy walking and appreciating the environment and to reap all the benefits of burning up more calories, toning your muscles, and energizing your body. Some people actually get paid for doing just that. Letter carriers who make door-to-door deliveries spend six hours or so walking every day and are compensated for it. Lumberjacks and construction workers may spend many hours each week walking.

You can incorporate what the construction worker and the letter carrier have in your life and reap something far more beneficial than monetary compensation: you can acquire the body and self-image that you desire.

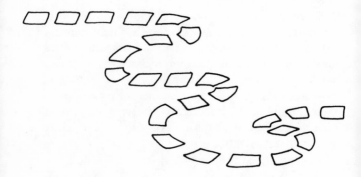

GET STARTED NOW

Start out by doing exercise that simply involves movement of your body through space. Begin being more active. Energize yourself rather than deplete your energy. Enjoy the activity and make it become part of your life-style. Rove in a city park where you can enjoy a stream or see dew on blades of grass. Watch butterflies in the spring; notice the frost in the winter. Hear children laugh and play, and watch the birds feed and then soar high into the sky to circle about again. Get in touch with the world.

Decide where roving will be enjoyable and listen to your body to find out how much roving is essential for your revitalization. Begin now. Stop reading at the end of this paragraph. Go for a stroll and make your plans.

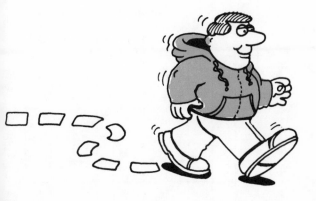

Daily Roving Record

Put a check mark in the box that shows the number of miles you roved. Try to reach the goals you set for yourself.

Beginning Date _____

MILES
ROVED

	First 7-day goal _____	Second 7-day goal _____	Third 7-day goal _____

10										
9½										
9										
8½										
8										
7½										
7										
6½										
6										
5½										
5										
4½										
4										
3½										
3										
2½										
2										
1½										
1										
½										
0										

1   3   5   7   9   11   13   15   17   19   21

restrict your grazing hours

Have you ever visited a midwestern dairy farm? If so, you will remember that the cows appear to graze all day. Many overweight people appear to do that, too. Others find that their harmful eating is restricted to a certain few hours of the day. They may not have a grazing problem during daylight hours because they have other things to occupy their minds. Since their Robot is not accustomed to eating while working, they find that the hours from six to eleven in the evening are the troublesome times. If your problem is restricted to those hours, it becomes easier to deal with.

In Chapter 8 you collected baseline data on your eating habits. You collected two kinds of data about time. One was how often and at what times of day you ate, and the second was how long you spent eating. Both data are helpful in building more effective habits.

The first thing you should do is study your baseline data and fill in the "Times When I Eat" column on the worksheet on page 124. You will note that this worksheet is divided into four columns: (1) Times When I Eat, (2) Unnecessary Times, (3) Sometimes Necessary Times, and (4) More Necessary Times.

In the Unnecessary column, put down the eating times that can be eliminated without too much trouble. For instance, we sometimes have a snack in the middle

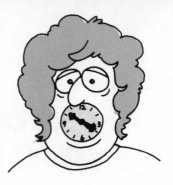

of the morning, such as a doughnut at coffee break. We can easily eliminate that snack by planning some creative option.

Other times are rather more necessary and more difficult to deal with. Social engagements may make eating seem more necessary to us. We might be able to skip a time when we normally eat if it is not surrounded with some kind of social activity. But when we sit down at a table with others, it seems appropriate to eat and difficult to avoid eating. These are the kinds of situations that we call "Sometimes Necessary."

Normally breakfast, lunch, and dinnertime make eating more necessary. In our culture we normally eat three times a day. The habit is often deeply engrained, so for most of us mealtimes are "Necessary" times.

Most dieters experience some especially difficult time. As we mentioned above, evening hours are often difficult times for overweight people.

DELETE UNNECESSARY TIMES

Look at the times when you eat unnecessarily, and plan a creative option. If you work in an office where the coffee break is a morning ritual of doughnuts and pastries, try to find an alternate activity. Get up and take a short walk or turn off the lights and relax for ten minutes while visualizing yourself as you approach

120

your weight goal. When you feel strong enough to pass up the doughnut, join the coffee break. Chew a piece of sugarless gum or have a cup of coffee with no sweetener. You should completely delete the least necessary times first.

TIMES THAT ARE SOMETIMES EASY TO DELETE

The third column lists times that are sometimes easy to delete. These times can be easily deleted part of the time, but at other times more effort is needed. Delete snacks or substitute an activity when you can. When you cannot, limit the size of the snack. Instead of eating three doughnuts or a 700-calorie meal, look ahead to your goal.

TIMES THAT I CANNOT DELETE

There are certain times of the day, usually mealtimes and occasionally special times, when it is extremely hard to simply delete eating situations. In cases like these you should try to develop healthier eating patterns.

Any overweight person can knock off a 1,200-calorie ham sandwich. Many can eat a 1,200-calorie sandwich right after dinner. If grazing in the evening is an especially difficult time for you, do not try to completely eliminate it at first. Instead, spend some time planning low-calorie options. Look at the list of low-calorie foods in Appendix I on page 190. If you normally finish dinner at six o'clock, plan to have a low-calorie snack around eight-thirty or nine. Avoid eating anything before your eight-thirty snack, and when you have it, make sure you plan carefully and make it attractive. Be sure that the portions are well measured and accurate.

When you are planning an optional snack, sit back, relax, and visualize just how it will look. Imagine yourself putting together a plate of low-calorie, high-fiber food. Make it a ritual. Sit down and enjoy the food—really enjoy it. Do not stand in front of the refrigerator and eat a cold hot dog. You can use the 180 calories that a hot dog represents to enjoy a really healthful snack.

WHEN YOU EAT TOO RAPIDLY

Eating too rapidly leads to overstuffing. Behavior modifiers work on the assumption that if the dieter eats more slowly, a feeling of satisfaction will be attained before the stomach is stuffed. Follow these rules:

1. Wait one full minute before starting to eat.
2. Place all food to be eaten on the plate before eating anything. Do not take second helpings.
3. Chew each bite and swallow it before placing more food in your mouth.
4. Put down silverware between each bite.
5. Make each meal last at least twenty minutes.

Slowing down can be achieved by practice. Before a meal, stop for a few moments and focus attention on the goal—to follow the rules.

PLAN FOR MORE JOY FROM LESS FOOD

The fifteen minutes before a meal is a crucial time to apply some of the techniques presented in previous chapters. It is a time to focus on the problem of your eating habits, to shift out of the Robot and take charge of your eating. If possible, sit down for ten minutes before you eat and focus your attention on the upcoming meal. Ask yourself if your Child is telling you that you really *need* this food, that unless you stuff yourself you are going to suffer anxiety and pain. Are you conducting a toxic internal dialogue? Yes, you do need to eat. But you do not need to eat everything in sight.

Relax, and visualize exactly what you are going to do when you eat. You are going to eat slowly; you are going to portion your food carefully; you are going to savor your times of eating and fully enjoy your food rather than stuffing it in.

Many people find that drinking a glass of ice water fifteen minutes before a meal helps curb the sensation of hunger. Try it and see if it works for you.

As you sit down to the meal, make sure you have some low-calorie, high-fiber food available—radishes, celery, and such like. Make sure, too, that you have some warm, low-calorie beverage to drink with your meal. Some people like a cup of bouillon; others enjoy unsweetened tea or coffee. Some people can drink just warm water. Focus on the sensation as you eat or as you drink a warm beverage. Most of all, enjoy this rational way of eating.

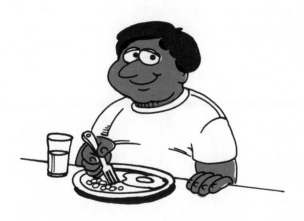

When Is Eating Really Necessary?

Fill in the blanks as accurately and as honestly as you can. Refer back to pages 119–120 for an explanation of what these "times" mean.

Times When I Eat	Unnecessary Times	Sometimes Necessary Times	More Necessary Times
_____	_____	_____	_____
_____	_____	_____	_____
_____	_____	_____	_____
_____	_____	_____	_____
_____	_____	_____	_____
_____	_____	_____	_____
_____	_____	_____	_____
_____	_____	_____	_____
_____	_____	_____	_____
_____	_____	_____	_____
_____	_____	_____	_____
_____	_____	_____	_____
_____	_____	_____	_____
_____	_____	_____	_____
_____	_____	_____	_____
_____	_____	_____	_____
_____	_____	_____	_____
_____	_____	_____	_____
_____	_____	_____	_____
_____	_____	_____	_____

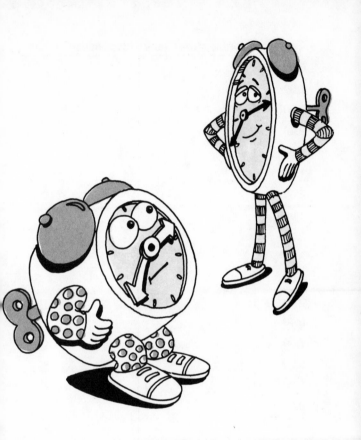

Building an Awareness of Times Linked to Eating

Most of us have particular times during the day when it seems especially difficult to resist eating. List your own difficult times. Then, from your list of options, plan some activity that will reduce the triggering cues and reinforce noneating.

125

	Troublesome Times	Activities/Options
6:00 a.m.		
7:00		
8:00		
9:00		
10:00		
11:00		
12:00		
1:00 p.m.		
2:00		
3:00		
4:00		
5:00		
6:00		
7:00		
8:00		
9:00		
10:00		
11:00		
12:00		
1:00 a.m.		
2:00		
3:00		
4:00		
5:00		
6:00		

Planning for Those Difficult Times

Most people have certain times and/or certain days when they are most likely to eat or snack between meals. Think about times when you have most difficulty eating sensibly (other than mealtimes), and list these times for each day of the week.

DAY	TIME	ACTIVITIES/OPTIONS
Monday		
Tuesday		

DAY	TIME	ACTIVITIES/OPTIONS
Wednesday		
Thursday		
Friday		

DAY	TIME	ACTIVITIES/OPTIONS
Saturday		
Sunday		

Now choose "good" activities from the Creative Options worksheet on pages 106–107 and write them in next to the "times." The more activities for each time, the better will be your options when you face these critical times.

This week, plan to involve yourself in your chosen activity during your critical times.

control the places where you eat

If you are a bona fide fatty, you will notice that you eat in hundreds of different places. You eat in the car, on the bus, in the bathroom, at the kitchen table, in front of the TV, while shopping, and so forth. The Robot loves that. It has learned to respond to eating cues in many different places. The goal of this chapter is to help you learn ways of restricting the areas in which you eat so as to restrict the eating cues for your Robot.

Take a look at Column 3 of your baseline data on pages 84–93. Under Step 1 of the worksheet on page 133, list *all* of the places where you ate during that ten-day period.

Under Step 2, list all the places that will be fairly easy for you to eliminate. Only you can be the judge of just where you can easily avoid eating. It may be in the car or when you're walking.

Under Step 3, list the more difficult places. A place is difficult to eliminate when we associate it with eating pleasure. For instance, when we go with the family to have an ice-cream cone, we eat in the car. Therefore the car is associated with pleasure because we enjoy the ice cream as well as the pleasure of being with the family.

Usually we can eliminate easy places without resorting to a reward system. We can simply cut them out.

Other places are rather more difficult to eliminate. Some overweight people have the deeply entrenched habit of standing by the sink and gobbling cookies or the last piece of cake. Housewives often have trouble eliminating tasting while they are cooking. They get in the habit of tasting all the foods they prepare whether they need to or not. These are rather more difficult habits to break. We probably need to apply some reward system as we eliminate those places.

Under Step 3 on the worksheet, make two columns. One should show places where you prefer to eat. Try to keep this number small. Most clinical behavior-modification programs focus on only one place. Your goal should be to reduce the number of places where you eat within your home to no more than two. Also, list the places that are not easy to eliminate but that you would like to eliminate. Since these are rather more difficult to eliminate, you may need to reward yourself or make use of creative options.

REWARD YOURSELF AS YOU BEGIN TO SUCCEED

Many behavior modifiers use a point system and a contract. Dieters keep precise records on how successful they are in moving toward a goal. For instance, if you set the goal of eliminating eating in the car, you

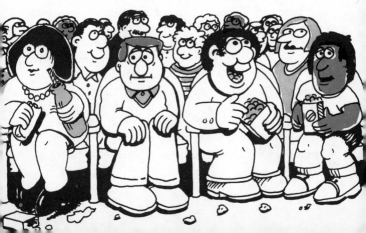

might give yourself five points each day you do not eat in the car. On a day when you did eat in the car, you would give yourself zero points. If at the end of the week you had more than twenty-five points, you would be due for a reward.

Some people respond to this system and feel it is very helpful in maintaining a high level of consciousness as to goals. Others do not respond well to such a mechanical procedure. The system you choose is not important. What *is* important is increasing your awareness of the unwanted eating habit and providing some reward when you successfully eliminate the habit.

Some people use money as a reward system. For instance, if you want to eliminate eating in the car, you might set aside a certain amount of money every day that you are successful. On days when you fall back into the old habit, no money is set aside or some is even removed from the kitty. The money, in a way, is its own reward, but it works better when you intend using it for something you would like to buy.

It is important to note that whatever reward you choose will fairly quickly lose its value. Points may work for a little while; money may work for a little while. But as soon as you begin to be bored with a reward, move to some new reward or system that will be genuinely satisfying.

Your aim should be to achieve two goals in your eating behaviors. One is the overall goal of reducing the number of calories in your total intake of food. The second is that of establishing effective and constructive eating habits. This can be accomplished by enhancing the occasions when you do eat. Try to make each meal a pleasant experience. Make the food look and taste good. Eat slowly. This latter is very important in reshaping eating behaviors. It is a way of reducing the number of cues that turns on your Robot eater.

Taking Control of Where We Eat

STEP 1	STEP 2	STEP 3	
All the Places Where I Eat	Places That Can Easily Be Eliminated	Places Difficult to Eliminate Would Like to Eliminate	Preferred
_____	_____	_____	_____
_____	_____	_____	_____
_____	_____	_____	_____
_____	_____	_____	_____
_____	_____	_____	_____
_____	_____	_____	_____
_____	_____	_____	_____
_____	_____	_____	_____
_____	_____	_____	_____
_____	_____	_____	_____
_____	_____	_____	_____
_____	_____	_____	_____
_____	_____	_____	_____
_____	_____	_____	_____
_____	_____	_____	_____
_____	_____	_____	_____
_____	_____	_____	_____
_____	_____	_____	_____
_____	_____	_____	_____
_____	_____	_____	_____

What rewards will I give myself as I succeed in eliminating unwanted habits?

_____

_____

How can I make eating more satisfying, less hurried, and more appropriate in the places where I choose to eat?

_____

_____

_____

_____

_____

eliminate triggering events

The cues that trigger eating behaviors vary greatly from person to person. After one session at the authors' workshops, a participant approached the director and asked how she was expected to lose weight when he wore a shirt with grapes printed on it. The grapes triggered hunger in her.

We all have some control over our environments— the places we go, the things that we choose to see in our environment. Since we have that modicum of control, we are free to eliminate some of the events that trigger eating behavior in us. Hunger pangs almost universally trigger eating behaviors, but many other internal sensations can also touch off eating. We have already seen that loneliness, fatigue, and anxiety often cause eating behaviors.

The time of the day is also often a trigger. That is why you have been asked to keep track of when you eat. Most of us have periods during the day when we find ourselves automatically drawn to the refrigerator. Eight o'clock, twelve o'clock, and six o'clock are regular mealtimes for many people in our culture, and those are very strong cues.

Social situations are still another typical trigger. We associate socializing with filling our faces because we almost always have food at parties and social gatherings.

Many people learn to eat when they do not feel well. Whether they are tired or feel a cold coming on, they act upon the general slogan, "Feed a cold, feed a fever, feed a rash, feed the heartbreak of psoriasis."

Visual and olfactory cues can also effectively trigger eating behaviors. Television commercials are particularly tempting. On Saturday morning children sit in front of the TV set and view all the junk-food commercials. By noon they have gobbled up your store of snack goods. Their eating behavior is triggered by the visual cues on TV.

There are other kinds of visual cues around the home. Most clinical programs of behavior modification strongly recommend that people cover all foods—that no food be left out in open containers where the dieter can easily see them. Some programs go so far as to suggest turning out the light in the refrigerator so that the food is not easily seen.

CLEAN UP YOUR ENVIRONMENT

As you look over your baseline data, you will see that there are quite a number of things that may trigger

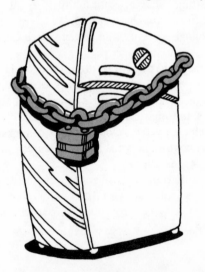

your eating behavior. Make a complete list of all the things you know trigger your automatic eating behavior. After you have made that list, note those that you can easily eliminate. Then do it. This may mean covering some foods and eliminating high-calorie snacks from your home.

There are other kinds of triggering events that you can eliminate only part of the time, such as social gatherings. When you go to a social gathering use one of the other tools, such as relaxation coupled with visualization.

LENGTHEN THE CHAIN

Psychologists talk about a chain of events leading up to a final behavior. Whenever we eat anything, there are some things we must do prior to the actual act of eating. If we have a cookie jar, the chain of events is a very short one. We walk into the kitchen, open the cookie jar, and eat the cookies. In unprepared foods, the chain is considerably longer. For instance, if we are to bake a cake from scratch, the chain is very long. If we buy a cake at a bakery, the chain is considerably shortened.

Behavior modifiers suggest that we lengthen the chain for foods that are inappropriate to our new lifestyle. Do not make cookies, cakes, and high-fat foods easily available. On the other hand, shorten the chain for low-calorie foods. Make them readily available. Keep a container of cleaned, ready-to-eat raw vegetables available in the refrigerator for those times when you feel compelled to eat. The long-term goal is, of course, to eliminate that in-between-meal eating.

On the next few pages are worksheets to help you recognize the things that trigger your eating. These exercises will enable you to develop creative options to replace the old automatic eating responses.

Building an Awareness of Events Linked to Eating

Events linked to eating are essentially those times and places which are likely to trigger eating. Examples are given in the left-hand column. List your own significant events in the right-hand column.

Examples of events that might trigger eating:	Rank order your events from "always" trigger eating to "seldom" trigger eating:
Eating out	1._____
Doing housework	2._____
Watching TV	3._____
Studying	4._____
Visiting	5._____
Entertaining	6._____
Idle Hours	7._____
Getting criticized	8._____
Movies	9._____
Parties	10._____
Insomnia	11._____
Cooking	12._____

Which are the easiest events for you to handle? What are the creative options which work best for you?

Events	Creative Options
1._____	_____
2._____	_____
3._____	_____

Once you succeed with these easiest events, pick a few more easy ones and decide on the best creative options for them. Remember to work on the easiest first, for it is with those that you are most likely to achieve success. Success will strengthen your motivation to tackle the more difficult events.

Building an Awareness of Feelings Linked to Eating

Most of us have associated eating (other than during mealtime) with certain feelings. Many people lose motivation for sensible eating when they are tired or lonely and are more susceptible to giving in to the urge to eat unless they have some viable or enjoyable options.

In the left-hand column are examples of feelings that might trigger overeating. List your own feelings in the right-hand column.

Examples of feelings that might trigger eating:	Rank order your feelings from "always" trigger eating to "may" trigger eating:
Bored	1._____
Anxious	2._____
Frustrated	3._____
Elated	4._____
Sad	5._____
Angry	6._____
Tired	7._____
Discouraged	8._____
	9._____
	10._____
	11._____
	12._____
	13._____
	14._____

Which are the easiest feelings for you to handle? What
are the creative options which work best for you?

Feelings   Creative Options

1._____   _____

2._____   _____

3._____   _____

Once you succeed with these easiest feelings, pick a
few more easy ones and decide on the creative options
which are most likely to succeed for you. Continue
working on this list until your life-style becomes one in
which feelings do not trigger eating.

PART THREE

ASSERTIVENESS AND WEIGHT CONTROL

A poet has said that no man is an island. He was not talking about the size people can attain, but rather the fact that we are social by our very nature.

We need each other. We especially need others when we set out to change our lives. Assertiveness can help us make and adjust our connections with other people.

ask for the help you need

Friends, relatives, and lovers can be an immense help in your program of personal growth and weight control. Research shows that the most successful approaches to building more effective eating patterns include educating those close to overweight people to give positive reinforcement. When close relatives or friends start rewarding overweight people for making progress rather than nagging and criticizing them for their inappropriate eating, the overweight people are well on their way toward learning new eating behaviors. Positive reinforcement leads to a positive self-image and good feelings about self rather than to self-hate and binge-inducing feelings.

Many people do not know how to express their needs or how to enlist the aid of others; they are easily discouraged and turned off by the comments of others. Weight control is a significant life change, and life changes seem to upset the feelings and behaviors of the people close to us. Attempts to change often bring negative or discounting reactions and unwanted attention to the overweight person. Such reactions are discouraging and stand between the overweight person and success in a weight-control program.

CHANGING RELATIONSHIPS IS SOMETIMES A THREAT

Overweight people are often subjected to discrimination in choice of schools, friendships, job opportunities, salary increases, and in other subtler ways. Did you ever try to find fashionable clothes when overweight? A tent is about as close as you can get to good-looking clothing.

In a way, overweight people are comfortable to be around because they provide no real competition. Slender people have the natural advantage, and because of this it may be in their interest to keep you fat. Their doing so may be unconscious, but you should be aware of this possibility.

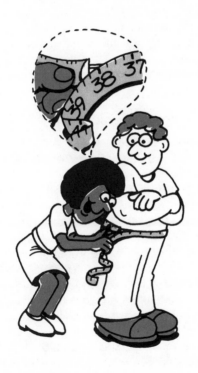

YOU HAVE A RIGHT TO WEIGHT CONTROL

The Declaration of Independence says everyone has the rights to life, liberty, and the pursuit of happiness. If losing weight is not the pursuit of happiness, nothing is. It may seem trite to even mention such basic rights, but experience shows that many overweight people feel that they have no rights because of their so-called weakness.

We all have the right to make basic decisions that affect our lives. Overweight people have the right to decide to take control of their eating habits.

It is important that you believe in your rights and that you act upon them. Until you assert your right to a healthy body, you will encounter a subtle resistance to your efforts to change. It is as though people are saying, "Get back in your place, fatty."

DO OTHER PEOPLE CONTROL YOUR EATING?

"You look *so* good the way you are."
"I had a friend who died from dieting."
"Have just a little—you can start tomorrow."
"What will the rest of the family do while you're dieting?"

Sometimes other people control us with subtle, and not so subtle, behavior. They push food at us. They disapprove when we do not eat as much as *they* think we should. They nag us when we leave a scrap of food and assume we are not serious in our efforts to change our lives. Many times they belittle our efforts to cut calories and eat healthier foods. They even presume to reassure us that the problem of being overweight is a genetic one and something we cannot change.

At times the people around us send the ulterior message that if we try to change, they will punish us by giving us the "cold shoulder." That strikes fear into the

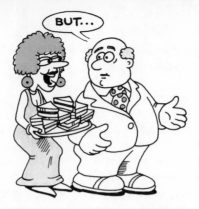

heart of a fatty. Rejection is the one thing that sends us to the consolation of the refrigerator.

There are three basic patterns of response to other people. These are described in the next few pages.

NONASSERTIVE BEHAVIOR SIMPLY DOES NOT WORK

Nonassertive individuals allow themselves to be bullied, directed, intimidated, led, and otherwise manipulated by others. They struggle all week to lose a pound, then overeat at a dinner party because the hostess thinks that overeating is a compliment and she "won't hear of you not eating all of that good dessert." The nonassertive overweight wife might forego buying low-calorie food because her husband has bullied her by teasing her about her diet.

In a technical sense, nonassertive behavior occurs whenever you let your rights be violated by others or when you violate your own rights by ignoring them. You are nonassertive when you ignore your right to be happy and healthy or when you let someone else direct you to do damaging things like overeating.

When you are nonassertive, you are emotionally dishonest, indirect, self-denying, and inhibited. You probably blame others for your overweight problem. When you act nonassertively, there are a number of unhappy consequences: You may feel hurt, anxious, and angry; then, you allow others to bully you, and you fail to generally achieve your desired goal of weight loss.

The nonassertive person wants to please others, but nonassertive behavior does not work that way. Other people may feel guilty or superior when you act nonassertively, or they may feel irritation, pity, or disgust.

Nonassertive behavior is a subtle type of manipulation. You give up your right to influence certain kinds of behavior—to eat correctly or make friends or avoid conflict—in the hope that others will notice and reward you. This kind of unspoken bargain seldom works because others generally take your self-sacrifice for granted. The nonasserter then ends up feeling bitter and cheated. In the language of Transactional Analysis, this is manipulation by the Victim.

Nonassertive behavior also spoils people around you by training them to think that they can make unreasonable demands on you and get away with it.

Nonassertive behavior also does not work because your true feelings are not expressed, and you carry them over into other situations. You might explode in anger and resort to eating binges at some later time.

AGGRESSIVENESS ON THE PART OF OTHERS

An aggressive person is one who bullies other people with threats and intimidation. In a technical sense, aggressiveness is interpersonal behavior in which people stand up for their own rights but violate the rights of others in the process. In the language of Transactional Analysis, it is the Persecutor role.

Aggressive behavior is an attack on the person rather than on the person's behavior. It is angry, hostile manipulation by blaming and intimidating others. This kind of behavior is emotionally dishonest because it is self-enhancing at the expense of others.

When people act aggressively, they may feel self-righteous and superior at the time, but guilty later. They achieve their desired goals by hurting others. They instill feelings of anger and vengeance in their victims.

More often than not, overweight people find themselves the target of aggressive behavior. Being overweight can often lead to feeling that we are weak and allowing ourselves to be bullied.

ASSERTIVE BEHAVIOR HELPS YOU ESTABLISH HELPFUL RELATIONSHIPS WITH OTHERS

When you act assertively, you take responsibility for your feelings and behaviors. This means that you can say no without feeling guilty. You can turn down food without offending the person offering it, and you can ask for the help you need when you need it.

Assertive behavior is standing up for your legitimate rights while respecting the rights of others. It enables you to act in your own best interests. It leads to a direct, honest, appropriate expression of your feelings, opinions, or beliefs. It shows consideration for but not deference to others. Assertive behavior is emotionally honest, direct, self-enhancing, and expressive.

BECOME MORE ASSERTIVE ABOUT LOSING WEIGHT

Assertiveness involves two things. First, it involves believing that you have the inalienable right to control your body and lose weight. Second, it involves practicing the skills of handling the "food pushers," disclosing to those closest to you your feelings and deep-set desire to lose weight, and asking for the support you need to repattern your behavior.

You have a right to be a healthy person—both physically and psychologically. When people say and do things that contribute to ill health, they are trampling on one of your most basic rights. You have no reason to allow yourself to be manipulated, and you certainly have no reason to feel guilty when you stand up for your rights.

Bolstered by your belief in your right to diet, you must still deal with people who consciously or unconsciously push food at you. First of all, do not try to justify or give reasons why you want to cut down. You *have* the right; you do not need to justify it. Second, when you turn down a snack, say no in a firm and definite voice, and repeat it as often as necessary to get the point across.

Tell the people closest to you just how important it is to you to rebuild your habits and lose weight. Do not expect thin people to fully understand your feelings. They probably cannot, anyway, because they have not had the experience. Do expect them to see the problem as much less crucial than you do. But do not play the victim. Just make the point that this diet is vital to your health, that you are serious about it, and that you want their support.

How do you ask for support? You just say, "This is a complex and difficult project and I need your support, not your criticism. Please notice my progress and comment on that." The next chapter is written for those people who are closest to you. Ask them to read it.

The following worksheet is designed to help you get in touch with your present level of assertiveness and to help you build assertive skills.

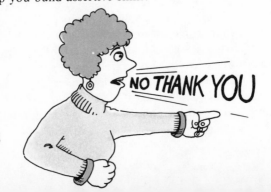

148

Assertiveness and Weight Control

We often feel compelled to eat, not out of hunger, but out of fear of hurting others' feelings. The following are somewhat typical examples of how others might try to tempt you. Put a check mark in the box that best expresses how you would probably respond.

	Would You Eat?		
	Yes	Maybe	No
1. "Have a piece of this cake—it's your favorite."	☐	☐	☐
2. "You aren't taking seconds. Didn't you like my cooking?"	☐	☐	☐
3. "Let's jump in the car and go get an ice-cream cone."	☐	☐	☐
4. "I don't like it when you diet because it changes our whole menu."	☐	☐	☐
5. "Our grocery bill increases whenever you go on a diet."	☐	☐	☐
6. "Put some Scotch in that club soda. I don't like drinking alone."	☐	☐	☐
7. "Here, take some more food; you can get back on your diet tomorrow."	☐	☐	☐
8. "Try some of this candy—it's delicious."	☐	☐	☐
9. "Can you finish the rest of this meatloaf? I hate to see it go to waste."	☐	☐	☐

	Would You Eat?		
	Yes	Maybe	No
10. "You aren't eating much. Is something wrong?"	☐	☐	☐
11. "Let's go to that smorgasbord restaurant for dinner."	☐	☐	☐
12. "Eat some more. I'm afraid you'll get sick if you don't eat more."	☐	☐	☐

You have the right to your privacy, and you can be private without offending others. Exercising that right is probably the easiest and best way to handle these situations. You do it by responding with brief one-liners: "I'm not hungry," "I'd rather not eat more," "I don't feel like having a drink," "Your cooking was great, but I'm full." Such one-liners permit you to close off prolonged discussion and argument about your reasons for not eating or drinking.

You may decide you want to go to an ice-cream parlor or eat at a smorgasbord restaurant, but you have the right to eat nothing. You might even join the crowd, have a low-calorie beverage, and enjoy everyone's company. If someone comments on your not eating, explain how important it is for you to stick with your diet. If that offends others, they either do not understand its importance to you or they are not concerned about what is good for you.

SOME FURTHER READING

Smith, M. J. *When I Say No, I Feel Guilty.* New York: Bantam, 1975. The author deals with the idea of assertiveness in clear and lucid prose. He outlines a number of assertive skills and shows, through sample dialogues, how they are applied.

a chapter for people who want to help

The fact that you are reading this means you are important to someone who is trying to lose weight and make some striking changes in his or her life. The first thing you must realize is that your response is far more important than you might think. You can help your friends lose weight in several ways and, in so doing, develop closer and happier relationships with them. Research shows that people trying to lose weight have far more success when their friends and family support them with positive comments about their successes. On the other hand, if you are negative in your attitude and impatient with the problems dieters face, you can be the final barrier to their success.

Losing weight is really two different problems. These problems are linked together and are often viewed as identical, but they are essentially different. One problem is simply the losing of excess weight accumulated over time. This is done by reducing food consumption to a level where the weight loser uses more energy than is taken in daily. The more overweight the person, the longer is the dieting period. The second problem is that the weight loser needs to repattern his or her eating habits. Habits are built up over a long period of time. Your help is needed to construct a systematic program that will change them.

Losing weight is very difficult for most people. For overweight people, food has become a symbol of comfort and security; removing or reducing the amount of food intake tends to provoke feelings of insecurity accompanied by psychological changes that make dieters grouchy and irritable.

BE PATIENT WITH ERRATIC BEHAVIOR

As people begin to diet, their behavior will tend to be rather erratic. Hunger, grouchiness, and discouragement can lead to eating binges. At those times, dieters should not be needled, but rather understood. The best thing you can do is be patient with such irrational behavior.

Dieters behave erratically because they have some irrational beliefs about themselves and about food. These beliefs were learned at a time when they were unable to sort things out and make them rational. They may have learned that they should always eat everything on their plate; when they fail to, they may feel guilty. The desire to lose weight conflicts with what they have learned, causing confusion and bad feelings.

Helping such people means getting them to restructure their environment. For instance, some dieters find it helpful to have someone else measure out their food.

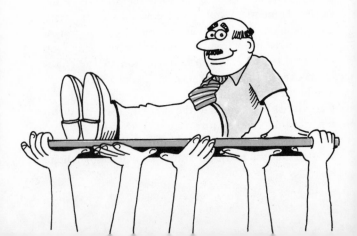

A reduction in the amount of high-calorie food available in the house may also be necessary.

LONELINESS AND FRUSTRATION OFTEN TRIGGER EATING

Overweight people often eat to satisfy feelings of loneliness, frustration, or boredom. This sets up a vicious circle. Negative feelings of frustration are often directly related to the dieters' overweight condition and their tremendous desire to lose that weight. The frustration itself triggers eating, and the eating increases the overweight problem. If you are working closely with dieters, it is very useful to become a good listener and try to encourage them to talk out their feelings of loneliness and frustration.

Dieters may be quite difficult to live with, especially during the early part of the dieting process. Try not to complain about the needed changes in life-style. A diet regimen may require you to stock up on high-protein, low-carbohydrate foods and reduce those that are high in calories. In the back of this book, on page 190, there is a list of foods that are especially good for dieting.

Eating is often triggered by certain items or events in the environment. A plate of cookies within easy reach can trigger mindless gobbling. You can help the weight loser by doing the following three things:

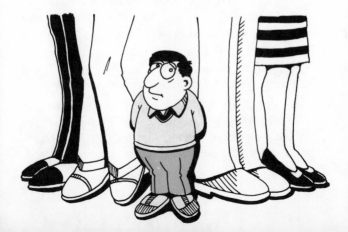

1. Clean the high-fat, high-carbohydrate foods out of the refrigerator and cupboards. Try not to make cookies, cakes, and pies easily available. Put other foods away in closed containers. Dieting is easier when food is not visible.
2. Make low-calorie substitutes easily available. Have plenty of raw vegetables and low-calorie beverages on hand, and encourage dieters to partake of them.
3. Help support the dieting process by encouraging new activities. The evening hours are often the hardest times for dieters. If possible, try to get dieters out of the house or apartment during those times. Suggest a walk. Encourage working on a hobby. Do whatever you can to keep dieters occupied.

Research shows again and again that praise and reward are very successful in helping people avoid frustration and maintain a positive outlook toward better eating habits. Two things motivate the dieter. One is weight loss itself. Another is a compliment from a friend or loved one. Sometimes dieters must go for days or weeks without any weight loss. So a word of encouragement can be a powerful incentive to stick with a diet.

Try not to complain about the changes dieters need to make in their life-styles. Do not nag about lack of progress or a temporary eating binge. Be encouraging at all times.

Finally, it is important to listen to the dieter. Try to be supportive of his or her weight-loss program.

A word of caution: Your part in this diet is to help your friend diet. You should not take the responsibility for the dieter's successes or failures. Part of the program is for the dieter to become increasingly self-reliant. Do not rescue; simply understand and encourage.

CHANGES IN A DIETER'S LIFE MEAN CHANGES IN YOURS

An interesting thing happens when people start to lose weight. As their bodies change, their relationships with people around them change somewhat. Overweight people are used to being treated differently than slim people. Others expect less of them in many ways; they do not offer much competition.

You may experience a feeling of anxiety as your dieting friends begin to change. Who knows where it comes from? Try to recognize it as the natural outcome of a changing relationship. Try to make the relationship grow. Be supportive. Help dieters achieve their goal and you will be building a positive, happier, and more intimate relationship.

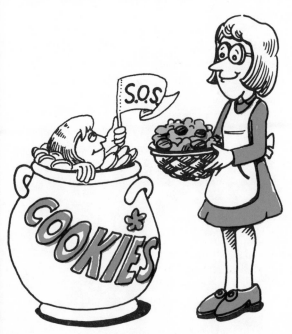

PART FOUR

A PRACTICAL MANUAL FOR WEIGHT CONTROL

This section presents some things you need to know about diets and calories. It also considers some topics that have been found to be of general interest to people in the authors' workshops.

a look at diets

Dr. Stillman; Weight Watchers; Dr. Atkins; Mayo; Computer; Prudent, Zen, and Cellulite diets; Boston Police Department, Vinegar-Kelp, B-6, or the Astronauts' diets: How does a person really interested in improving overall health and losing weight make sense of all these diets?

The study of nutrition has been around for quite some time. We have all studied the basic food groups in school. But some questions remain, perhaps many. How can we make sense of our nutritional needs? What are the basic principles that we must follow in order to have a truly healthful diet? Can we reduce our food intake and still be healthy? How much fat do we need? Should we eliminate carbohydrates?

The modern diet tends to be sufficient in calories but often contains too much sugar, fat, cholesterol, and salt. Each of these elements plays an important role in nutrition, but when taken in excess they are troublesome and often lead to serious physical disability.

William Dufty wrote a book called *Sugar Blues*. In it he talks about how sugar has become an important factor in the diets of most people in the Western world. He goes to great lengths to trace the history of sugar and links it with many degenerative diseases, primarily obesity and diabetes.

There is no doubt that most of us have a far greater concentration of sugar in our diet than is really healthful. Nutritionists agree upon that. It harms our teeth and provides calories that are basically void of nutritional value. One principle of improved diet generally recognized by nutritionists is that we can achieve a better diet by reducing our intake of sugar.

American diets contain far too much fat. This is probably an outcome of the affluence of this country. We eat large quantities of meat; and while meat contains high levels of protein, it also contains high levels of fat. Worse than that, meat generally contains saturated fat that is linked to atherosclerosis and heart disease. In the past ten years it has been shown that when the amount of fat in the diet is reduced, and polyunsaturated fats are substituted for saturated fats, the incidence of atherosclerosis and heart disease is also reduced. The second principle, then, is to reduce the total amount of fat in our diets.

Cholesterol is an element that is needed and utilized within the body, but when taken in excess it is linked with heart disease. So a healthful diet limits the amount of cholesterol ingested. The third principle is to limit the amount of cholesterol in our diet.

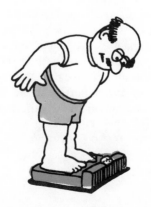

Sodium is linked to hypertension, or high blood pressure, and salt is the primary source of sodium in the diet. Nutritionists estimate that most Americans eat ten times as much salt as is needed to maintain a healthful, balanced diet. So a fourth principle of a healthful diet is to reduce the amount of salt.

THE TOP DIET

Jean Mayer describes a healthful diet in his book, *Overweight: Causes, Cost and Control.* He says: "A diet which gives you a relatively large proportion of protein; no more than 30% of fat, with unsaturated fat predominant; and a minimum of carbohydrates (no less than 60 grams) and very little sugar, is the best diet."* Well, that just about describes a good diet in a very brief way.

That is a rather technical description of nutrition, and it may be difficult for many people to understand. What does it mean? Probably the best way to answer that question is to describe the highest-rated diet as chosen by *Consumer's Guide* in the book, *New Ways to Lose Weight . . . Rating the Diets.* In that publication, the New York City Department of Health diet was rated as the very top. A copy of that diet appears on the following pages.

This book has been primarily concerned with the psychological war on fat. It has made an attempt to present ways of dealing with your feelings and modifying your behavior so as to develop better eating habits and become healthier—both psychologically and physically. The aim has not been to provide nutritional data or diets. It is important, however, that you see an example of a nutritionally satisfying, realistic, limited-calorie diet.

---

*Jean Mayer, *Overweight: Causes, Cost and Control* (Englewood Cliffs, N.J.: Prentice-Hall, 1968), p. 160.

Eat to Lose Weight

The New York Health Department Diet

For Most Women and Small Frame Men

BREAKFAST
High Vitamin C Fruit
  Choose ONE from "Food Facts"
Protein Food—Choose ONE:
  2 oz. cottage or pot cheese
  1 oz. hard cheese
  2 oz. cooked or canned fish
  1 egg
  8 oz. cup skimmed milk
Bread or Cereal, whole grain or enriched—
Choose ONE:
  1 slice bread
  ¾ cup ready-to-eat cereal
  ½ cup cooked cereal
Coffee or Tea

LUNCH
Protein Food—Choose ONE:
  2 oz. fish, poultry or lean meat
  4 oz. cottage or pot cheese
  2 oz. hard cheese
  1 egg
  2 level tablespoons peanut butter
Bread—whole grain or enriched—2 slices
Vegetables—raw or cooked—except potato
  or substitute
Fruit—1 serving
Coffee or Tea

DINNER
Protein Food—Choose ONE:
  4 oz. cooked fish, poultry or lean meat
Vegetables—cooked and raw
  High vitamin A—Choose from "Food Facts"
  Potato or Substitute—Choose ONE from
    "Food Facts"
  Other Vegetables—you may eat freely
Fruit—1 serving
Coffee or Tea

Other Daily Foods:
Fat—Choose 3 from "Food Facts"
Milk—2 cups (8 oz. each) skimmed or substitute from
  "Food Facts"

Food Facts

LIMIT THESE PROTEIN FOODS

Lean beef, pork, lamb to 1 pound per week total

Eggs to 4 per week
Hard cheese to 4 oz. per week

HIGH VITAMIN C FRUITS (No added sugar)

1 medium Orange
½ medium Cantaloupe
1 cup Strawberries
½ medium Mango

4 oz. Orange/Grapefruit juice
½ medium Grapefruit
1 large Tangerine
8 oz. Tomato juice

OTHER FRUITS (No added sugar)

1 medium Apple or Peach
1 small Banana or Pear
¼ lb. Cherries or Grapes
½ cup Pineapple
½ cup Berries

2-3 Apricots/Prunes/Plums
½ round slice Watermelon
  (1" by 10")
½ small Honeydew Melon
2 Tablespoons Raisins

HIGH VITAMIN A VEGETABLES

Broccoli	Mustard greens, Collards,	Spinach
Carrots	and other leafy greens	Watercress
Chicory	Pumpkin, Winter Squash	Escarole

POTATO OR SUBSTITUTE

1 medium Potato
1 small Sweet Potato
  or Yam
½ cup cooked Rice
Spaghetti, Macaroni,
  Grits or Noodles

1 small ear Corn
½ cup Corn or green
  Lima Beans, Peas
½ cup cooked dry
  beans, Peas, Lentils

FAT

1 teaspoon Vegetable Oil
1 teaspoon Mayonnaise
2 teaspoons French
  Dressing

1 teaspoon Margarine
  with liquid vegetable oil
  listed first on label
  of ingredients

SKIMMED MILK OR SUBSTITUTE

2 cups (8 oz. each) Buttermilk
1 cup (8 oz.) Evaporated Skimmed Milk
2/3 cup nonfat Dry Milk Solids

For Most Men and Large Frame Women

BREAKFAST

High Vitamin C Fruit
  Choose ONE from "Food Facts"
Protein Food—Choose ONE:
  2 oz. cottage or pot cheese
  1 oz. hard cheese

2 oz. cooked or canned fish
1 egg
8 oz. cup skimmed milk
Bread or Cereal, whole grain or enriched—Choose ONE:
   2 slices bread
   1½ cups ready-to-eat cereal
   1 cup cooked cereal
Coffee or Tea

LUNCH

Protein Food—Choose ONE:
   2 oz. fish, poultry or lean meat
   4 oz. cottage or pot cheese
   2 oz. hard cheese
   1 egg
   2 level tablespoons peanut butter
Bread—whole grain or enriched—2 slices
Vegetables—raw or cooked—
   except potato or substitute
Fruit—1 serving
Coffee or Tea

DINNER

Protein Food—Choose ONE:
   6 oz. cooked fish, poultry or lean meat
Vegetables—raw and cooked
   High Vitamin A—Choose from "Food Facts"
   Potato or Substitute—Choose ONE from "Food Facts"
   Other vegetables—you may eat freely
Fruit—1 serving
Coffee or Tea

OTHER DAILY FOODS

Fat—Choose 6 from "Food Facts"
Milk—2 cups (8 oz. each) skimmed or
      substitute from "Food Facts"

YOU MAY DRINK—

Coffee	Water	Bouillon
Tea	Club soda	Consomme

YOU MAY USE—

Salt	Herbs	Lemon, Lime
Pepper	Spices	Vinegar
	Horseradish	

YOU MAY EAT FREELY—

Asparagus	Cucumber	Romaine
Green Beans	Dandelion	Lettuce
Broccoli	Greens	Spinach

Brussels Sprouts	Escarole	Summer
Carrots	Kale	Squash
Cauliflower	Lettuce	Swiss Chard
Celery	Mushrooms	Tomato
Chicory	Mustard Greens	Turnip Greens
Collards	Parsley	Watercress

YOU MAY NOT EAT OR DRINK—

Bacon, Fatty Meats, Sausage	Gelatin Desserts, Puddings (sugar-sweetened)
Beer, Liquor, Wines	Gravies and Sauces
Butter, Margarines other than described in "Food Facts"	Honey, Jams, Jellies, Sugar and Syrup
Cakes, Cookies, Crackers, Doughnuts, Pastries, Pies	Ice Cream, Ices, Ice Milk, Sherbets
Candy, Chocolates, Nuts	Milk, Whole
Cream—Sweet and Sour, Cream Cheese, Non-Dairy Cream Substitutes	Muffins, Pancakes, Waffles
	Olives
French Fried Potatoes, Potato Chips	Soda (sugar-sweetened)
Pizza, Popcorn, Pretzels and Similar Snack Foods	Yogurt (fruit-flavored)

THIS IS YOUR DIET
THE REST IS UP TO YOU

SOME FURTHER READING

Berland, Theodore. *New Ways to Lose Weight . . . Rating the Diets.* Skokie, Ill.: *Consumer Guide*, 1976. This book gives the pros and cons of a large number of diets. The descriptions are clear and concise—an excellent starting point when looking at diets.

Dufty, W. *Sugar Blues.* New York: Warner, 1976. The author presents a historical-to-contemporary use of sugar in our diets and indicates the health problems associated with high sugar intake. Of special note to dieters is his conclusion that large intakes of sugar will increase appetite and hunger.

Mayer, J. *A Diet for Living.* New York: Pocket Books, 1977. A book that thoroughly covers nutrition, that is, proteins, fats, carbohydrates, vitamins, and minerals. The author recommends a nutritionally sound lifelong diet from toddlerhood to old age. He relates weight to well-being through proper eating and exercise. Helpful ideas on buying and preparing foods are also given.

———. *Overweight: Causes, Cost and Control.* Englewood Cliffs, N.J.: Prentice-Hall, 1968. The author covers the topics of hunger, obesity, and disease. He discusses genetics and obesity, activity and weight control, social attitudes regarding overweight, the psychology of obesity, and science and nutrition.

balancing energy

In the final analysis, the many approaches to dieting all rely upon the same principle. It goes something like this. Body fat is stored energy. That stored energy is drawn from the foods we eat and drink. Most of the foods we eat are used as fuel to keep our bodies warm and to enable us to move about. The colder it is and the more we move about, the more energy we use. The more energy we use, the more food we need. However, when the food we eat contains *more* energy than we need to heat our bodies and generate energy, that excess energy *is stored as fat*. That works two ways. If we take in *less* food than needed for warmth and energy, the excess energy needed is taken from the stored fat in our bodies. It is very simple—calories do count. If we eat *more* than we use up, we put on weight; if we eat *less* than we use up, we lose weight. Everyone has some body fat. Some of us simply have too much.

SOME DIETS CLAIM TO BE QUICKER THAN OTHERS

A number of diets are designed to provide quick weight losses right at the beginning. These diets are based on the idea that a quick weight loss encourages the dieter. Once the quick weight loss is achieved, the person will be motivated to continue with the diet.

Most of the quick diets operate on one of two principles. One, they reduce the amount of salt intake, or they provide some diuretic such as vitamin C; this magnifies the normal weight loss by causing the body to shed some of its stored water. Second, they severely restrict the amount of calories eaten.

Many nutritionists argue that in the long run quick diets are nutritionally unsound. They note, and rightly so, that quick weight loss as a result of water loss is not a loss of true fat. As soon as the diet is over, the weight comes back immediately.

SOME DIETS DO NOT DIRECTLY COUNT CALORIES

A number of diets use as a selling point the fact that they do not involve counting calories. The New York City Department of Health diet and the Weight Watchers diet do not mention calories. There are certain other "exchange" diets that claim there is no need to count calories. This is only partly true. What the builders of these diets are really saying is that if you are willing to *measure* your food, you do not have to count calories. The nutritionists who specified the portions have already counted the calories for you. The dieter counts calories by measuring.

People with a weight problem must understand the basic idea of calorie counting. At some time we all want to get off the restrictions of this or that diet and eat some (not all) of our favorite foods. We long for the foods we like, and we need to know how to eat those foods in quantities that will help us either continue to lose weight or maintain weight. The only way this can be done is by calorie counting. A complete calorie counter is supplied at the end of this book in Appendix II beginning on page 191.

WHAT IS A CALORIE?

A calorie is a measure of energy. It relates to the amount of energy it takes to warm up a given quantity of water. The important thing to note is that a pound of fat is made up of 3,500 calories. Translated into very simple terms, this means that if your intake of food is 500 calories *less* than what you burn up each day, you will lose an average of one pound per week. Similarly, if your intake is 500 calories *more*, you will add one pound per week.

How many calories do you need to maintain your weight? The following chart answers that question. First, locate your weight in the column at the far left. Next, choose the description of how active you are. In order to compute this, think of what you do on an hour-by-hour basis. Decide which column you should use. Then, look at the number of calories in that column opposite your weight. That will give you the number of calories you need per day to maintain your weight. You can then compute an effective diet by subtracting either 500 or 1,000 calories from your weight-maintenance number, depending on whether you want to lose one or two pounds per week.

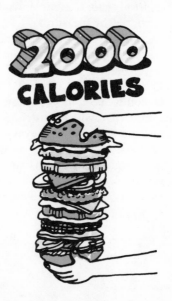

Your Activity and the Use of Calories

YOUR Weight	Your weight-maintenance number when you are very inactive (your weight multiplied by 12).	Your weight-maintenance number when you are medium active (your weight multiplied by 16).	Your weight-maintenance number when you are very active (your weight multiplied by 20).
95	1140	1520	1900
101	1212	1616	2020
110	1320	1760	2200
120	1440	1920	2400
130	1560	2080	2600
140	1680	2240	2800
150	1800	2400	3000
160	1920	2560	3200
175	2100	2800	3500
185	2220	2960	3700
195	2340	3120	3900
200	2400	3200	4000
210	2520	3360	4200
220	2640	3520	4400
230	2760	3680	4600
240	2880	3840	4800

TROUBLE SHOOTING IN CALORIE COUNTING

One of the constant complaints heard from overweight people is that they are on a 1,200-calorie diet but are not losing weight. In most cases this is attributable to two phenomena. One is what nutritionists call a "plateau." After a significant weight loss, the body goes through a period of readjustment. Chapter 19 deals with this phenomenon. The best advice to those on a plateau is to stick with the diet and be assured that good weight loss will recur soon.

The second cause is that unwanted and unrecorded calories start popping back into the diet. This is the most common reason for slowed weight loss. People do several things that cause them to misjudge the amount of food they eat. They may eat small quantities but fail to record the calories in those small snacks. If they snack several times during the day, the calories add up quickly but remain unnoticed. Enough calories are added to prevent weight loss.

Sometimes people have the strange idea that if food doesn't taste good or if it is liquid, the calories do not count. As was mentioned before, two glasses of orange juice contain as many calories as a medium-sized breakfast.

Sometimes people fail to realize how many calories are contained in certain kinds of foods. Fats and oils are very high in calories—nine calories per gram compared to five calories per gram for carbohydrates and proteins. So any food that contains a high proportion of fats or oils will tend to be very high in calories. Even a small snack that is high in fats or oils adds up tremendously.

One of the authors thought he could stay on a diet by snacking on soybeans at lunchtime and otherwise skipping meals. After a couple of weeks, he was shocked to find out that soybeans contain almost 700 calories per cup and that he was, in fact, taking in 300 to 500 more calories than he thought he was. Nuts, seeds, meats, and a few fruits like avocado contain a high proportion of fats. These foods are to be avoided.

Sometimes, too, we count our calories but fail to count the "extras." Often these extras are more fattening than the basic dish itself. It is one thing to eat a medium-sized baked potato. It is another thing to eat a baked potato oozing with sour cream or butter.

Calorie counting, then, is based on a simple process: (1) we need to know the calorie content of the food we are eating, (2) we need to know the quantities of food

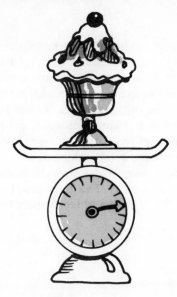

that we are consuming, and (3) we need to keep close track of the number of calories contained in the foods we eat. We need to record *all* the foods we eat. Appendix III contains a chart where you can record your daily calorie consumption.

CONTINUOUS EATING

Many people have little idea of how much food they eat because of their particular style of eating. They eat second and third helpings without even realizing it. They actually lose track of how much food they eat. One of the authors had a good friend who continually claimed that she ate next to nothing, yet she maintained an unhealthy load of fat. This was puzzling for some time until the author saw her at a party. She stood by the buffet table and continually added quantities of food to her plate before it was empty. The total amount of food consumed was obviously enough to maintain her obese condition, but she was genuinely unaware of just how much she was eating.

171

If you have that kind of problem, follow a couple of simple rules. First, measure your food accurately. Make sure that your three-ounce patty of hamburger is three ounces, not five ounces. Second, put all the food you plan to eat on your plate. Do not go back for seconds. If you feel your diet would permit a small second helping of some item, be sure to eat all of the food on your plate before taking it.

Many people have found it psychologically beneficial to use smaller plates. This gives the appearance of a larger quantity of food and seems more satisfying.

the infernal plateau

All dieters have experienced a leveling-off in their weight-loss pattern. You go on a diet; you lose weight regularly for a few weeks; then, even while staying on the diet, you find that for a week or more there is no weight loss at all. You may even gain a pound or two. This has come to be known as a "plateau" among people in weight-loss programs.

A plateau can be terribly discouraging. Eating and overeating are rewarded by the taste of food and the feelings accompanied by a full stomach. Weight loss is the primary reinforcer for most people trying to lose weight. So when weight loss stops, it is very difficult to maintain motivation to continue dieting.

WHAT CAUSES A PLATEAU?

There are a number of things that can cause a plateau. The most likely cause is related to the fact that the loss of fat is not the same thing as the loss of weight. Certain factors influence the loss of weight, primarily the retention of water. This is especially true in women. Because of their hormonal structure, women tend to retain more water during certain phases of their menstrual cycle. The retention of water is influenced in both men and women by the amount of sodium ingested. The primary source of sodium is salt. So the more salt we eat in our food, the more water we will retain in our bodies.

During a plateau there is often a continued loss in body *fat* but a temporary cessation of the loss of *weight*, because the loss of fat is more than compensated for by the retention of more water.

The authors often tell people to avoid weighing themselves the day after they go to a restaurant. Restaurant food is apt to be high in sodium content. Even after a relatively low-calorie meal, many people will put on a little weight the following day. It is a temporary weight gain. A gain in water is not a gain in fat.

SOME OTHER REASONS FOR THE PLATEAU

Another reason for the leveling-off in weight loss is a loss of motivation as we become satisfied with our progress. Because of the lower motivation, we allow more high-calorie foods back into our diet. This is especially true when we move away from a rigid diet and begin making substitutions. As we introduce foods into our diet that are high in fat or salt, we find that our weight loss is curtailed severely.

Diminishing motivation also comes about because friends no longer tend to notice how well we are doing. As we begin to enjoy success and as dieting becomes a routine, people notice us less and give us fewer strokes as a result. This causes our motivation to diminish.

Take heart when you are on a plateau. It is a natural occurrence during most diets. Do not fall back into toxic self-talk. Tell yourself the truth: This is temporary. You can compensate by reducing the amount you eat for a couple of days.

DEALING WITH THE PLATEAU

Patience is probably the key virtue in dealing with plateaus; however, patience is the thing that overweight people are very short of. Even though it took us

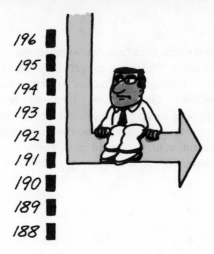

196
195
194
193
192
191
190
189
188

years to accumulate our excess fat, we are always in a hurry to get rid of it. But patience is more than a virtue. It is an Adult way of relating to some rather natural processes. The opposite of patience is discouragement, and discouragement is something that comes out of our Child. Our Child wants to use the plateau as an excuse to stuff ourselves and jump back into that vicious circle.

Spend some of the time on the plateau reflecting on your successes. You have lost some weight; you have begun to feel better about yourself; you can see that success is within your grasp. Think like a winner. Put the diet back into the forefront of your consciousness by reaccumulating baseline data. Spend some time analyzing your self-talk and dealing with your feelings.

Restructure your rewards. Rewards work for only a relatively short time. Try to find new things with which to reward your successes—things that you will be excited about and that will maintain your concentration. Go back and reread the chapter on "Psychological Tools and Creative Options."

At this point you are ready to read some things other than diet literature. Pick up some self-help books on interpersonal relationships. Practice assertive skills. Make a new friend. Get to know your family better. While maintaining dieting as a priority, try to move away from a preoccupation with food and dieting and begin to expend your energy in new, positive, and productive ways. Before you know it, you will be off the plateau.

CHAPTER **20**

coping with binges

Many dieters are haunted by eating binges. An eating binge is compulsive or unscheduled eating behavior. It is usually attended by strong feelings and the "need" to stuff oneself. Dieters often think of a binge as uncontrollable behavior. While such behavior is difficult to deal with, it is by no means uncontrollable.

Any one of several things can be happening to a person who feels a binge coming on. Perhaps the diet no longer has priority in the consciousness of the dieter. This may be because dieting is a priority in the Adult ego state while hunger and irrational behavior still exist in the Child ego state. In a way it might be said that the hungry Child is getting the upper hand.

"Binging" behavior is often triggered by feelings of self-pity, anxiety, anger, or frustration. The Child has learned to deal with those feelings by indulging in pleasure as compensation.

THE PROBLEM IS STOPPING IT

The best thing to do when you feel an eating binge coming on is to remove yourself as far as possible from your immediate environment. Get out of the house or apartment; go for a walk; involve yourself in some completely different and enjoyable activity. Choose an option that is not linked with food. Get involved in your hobby. Work in a darkroom. Knit, paint, read, or practice a musical instrument.

Once you have interrupted the "binging" behavior, spend time reorganizing your priorities. Shift back into the Adult ego state and list all of the reasons why you want to lose weight and why overeating is inappropriate behavior. When you go on a binge, you move from the personal-growth circle back into the vicious circle of increasing your weight and feeling discouraged about it. You know that reducing your food intake will make you happier and healthier, and that going on a binge will ultimately make you feel terrible.

IF YOU CANNOT AVOID THE BINGE, LIMIT IT

Sometimes it is very difficult to remove yourself from the environment that triggers eating behavior; other times you may have nagging problems that just will not dissipate easily. If this is the case, limit the binge. You can do this in several ways.

First of all, do not rush into the binge. Before you eat, examine your self-talk and try to put yourself on a positive track. Go to the calorie listings in Appendix I on page 190 and choose some of the foods that are low or moderate in calories, such as vegetables. Cook your-

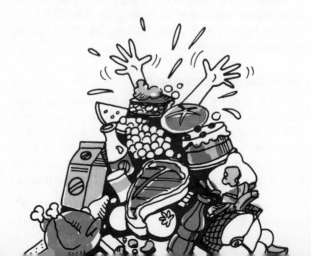

self some green beans or mushrooms, both of which are low in calories. Eat only food that you prepare and that is warm when you eat it. Warm food is more satisfying.

Put your food on a small plate and eat slowly. Enjoy the food and try to limit it. While you are eating, generate positive self-talk. Tell yourself how much progress you have made since the times when you used to stuff yourself with high-calorie foods and then felt depressed.

TALK TO A FRIEND

Many people like the approach developed by Alcoholics Anonymous. When they feel the old behaviors coming on, they immediately go to the phone and talk with someone who is familiar with the behaviors and who has experienced similar kinds of problems. Talking with other people often makes us feel better and removes the triggering event. Sometimes talking can help us eliminate the binge completely.

People also find that reading a book about nutrition or dieting is helpful. Being in touch with those who are concerned and knowledgeable about diets is often a helpful way of reducing the impulse to eat in an uncontrolled way.

RELAXATION MAY HELP

In the chapter, "Psychological Tools and Creative Options," we talked about relaxation and meditation as tools to be used in dealing with eating habits. Eating binges are often attended by anxiety and a general inability to concentrate on one thing at a time. Relaxation is an excellent approach to reducing that physical discomfort.

When you feel a binge coming on, find a place where you can sit back, relax, and go through the steps of deep relaxation. This will reduce your anxiety, and it will give you a chance to reestablish your priorities and shift ego states.

WHAT YOU TELL YOURSELF IS CRUCIAL

Many people tell themselves in their internal dialogue that they cannot control their behavior when they are on an eating binge. This is very toxic self-talk, and it reinforces the "binging" pattern of behavior. Try telling yourself the truth. Tell yourself that you are anxious or unhappy or very hungry and that you are trying to compensate by stuffing yourself. That is learned behavior. Since you are an intelligent adult, you can change that learned behavior.

Tell yourself that a binge does not really help you. It involves you in that vicious circle where your feelings will not be improved in the long run but will, in fact, get worse. Your physical condition will get worse, and your feelings about yourself will get worse.

To recapitulate, there are three ways to cope with binges. First, get away from the situation or the feelings that trigger the "binging" behavior. Second, if the former is completely impossible, limit the binge. Eat some satisfying low-calorie foods. Put away everything else, and do not allow yourself more than a certain amount of food. When you begin to feel better and more satisfied, stop eating. You *can* stop in the middle of a binge, and the sooner you stop, the better. Third, when you are on a binge, try to concentrate on the things that you are telling yourself. Say positive, powerful, enhancing things instead of killer statements such as, "I'm completely out of control" or "I can't handle my own life."

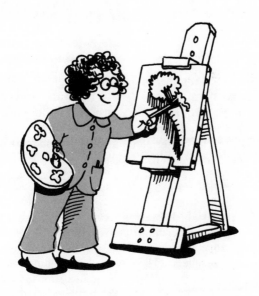

some questions and answers

There are a number of questions people characteristically ask the authors in their workshops. Some of the more popular questions are answered in this chapter. The questions and answers have been limited to those related to the material in this book and make no attempt to provide nutritional specifics or recommend particular diets.

1. Are weight-loss groups effective?

We are social animals. Historically we have banded together to satisfy our needs and solve our problems. The majority of us gain incentive and motivation by belonging to an organized group such as TOPS, Weight Watchers, or Overeaters Anonymous, or by forming our own neighborhood groups.

Many people find comfort in sharing a common problem and are motivated to succeed in weight-loss groups. One important element in group approaches is that usually some financial investment must be made to gain membership. Research indicates a greater likelihood of success if we must make some investment and commitment. Therefore, the money and time are usually well worth it.

2. What about the use of appetite suppressants or diet pills?

The American public annually spends millions of dollars ($80 million in 1969) for appetite suppressants. This reflects the severity of the problem of obesity and the urgency with which people desire to shed pounds.

There may be benefits to appetite suppressants. Some people have lost pounds by following over-the-counter diet plans or by using prescribed diet pills. The pitfall is that if the plan works, we are tempted to credit our weight loss to the diet plan or pill rather than to ourselves. This book is directed toward crediting yourself, enhancing your personal growth and self-esteem. Dependence on pills is contrary to that intent. You must ultimately make the decision about appetite suppressants. Will they enhance you or rob you of self-fulfillment?

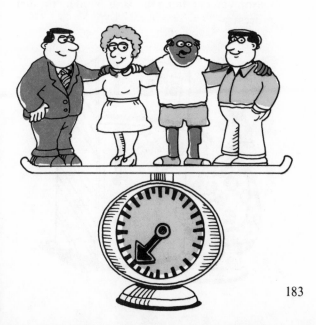

3. How do I maintain motivation?

That is probably the most often-asked question. Review Chapter 9, "Psychological Tools and Creative Options." Try to find ways of keeping your diet a priority in your life. You can do this by setting attainable goals, visualizing success, maintaining positive self-talk, and interrupting a binge by removing yourself from temptation.

To remain motivated means to remind yourself that the diet is a priority for you. We often make the mistake of not bringing our goals to mind throughout the day. Create ways to remind yourself of the importance of your diet. The reminders need to be changed often to maintain their effectiveness. Reminders may be things like notes on the refrigerator door or a small piece of tape on your watchband reminding you of your diet. While you rove or exercise, recall that the reason you are doing this is to speed up the diet process.

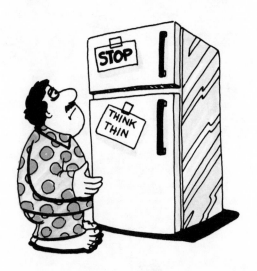

4. How do I stay on a diet when I have social commitments or am entertaining?

Preplanning is the key. Anticipate what will happen by imagining the social situation. For example, relax prior to a social engagement and vividly imagine yourself in that situation. Think of what willpower and self-control you will show, and visualize yourself eating very moderate portions.

Social situations generate social anxiety, and the diet may lose its priority. When social anxiety takes priority, you will do almost anything to become more comfortable. That probably includes eating and drinking. By preplanning and visualizing the occasion, you will be prepared to be calm, relaxed, and able to enjoy the social situation without overindulging.

5. I have the habit of tasting things when I cook. How can I break that habit?

There are at least two approaches that work well. First, know how many calories you consume with each taste so that you can count that in on your total daily calorie intake. Second, use behavior modification to lessen or eliminate the tasting. You would only choose the first alternative if you felt that you could not cook well without tasting the meal during preparation.

Most people can prepare a meal without tasting it at certain stages of development. If you choose not to taste your cooking, be sure to set up a reward system for avoiding the temptation. Meal preparation often comes at a time when the cook is hungry. One way around that is to prepare the meal in advance, right after an earlier meal. Another approach is to reward yourself with something you wanted to do or buy or see if you can successfully prepare meals for two days without sampling the food as you prepare it.

6. I wake up one or two hours after having gone to bed and am very groggy and hungry. How do I keep myself from going to the refrigerator and cleaning it out?

People who tend to "sleep-eat" usually munch on snack foods. This means you need to clean up your environment in order to break the habit. It is unlikely that you would spend forty-five minutes in the middle of the night preparing a dish. So you should remove snack items such as nuts, cookies, apple pie, and ice cream. Another alternative is to prepare a low-calorie snack such as carrot sticks or celery prior to bedtime; eat only that, and return to bed.

7. How important is exercise to dieting and a proper life-style?

As you begin dieting, increase your exercise moderately. For most overweight people, active exercise such as jogging is unappealing. However, many people enjoy a stroll through a park or a short walk around the block or around their own yard.

"Roving" is recommended because almost everyone can comfortably walk a reasonable distance. Find your own limits. A walk that exhausts you is too far. A walk that invigorates you is your appropriate limit.

Once you have found your appropriate limit, set goals to increase that limit. If you can comfortably walk one block, you should be walking two blocks by the second week. If at present you can easily walk a mile, try walking two miles and increasing that. Experts say that walking ten miles a day is a healthy amount of exercise.

8. What about fasting?

We know from history that human beings can live long periods of time on very poor diets. The concentration camps during World War II showed some of the long-term results. There were tremendous weight losses from malnutrition, and many victims died.

Most nutritionists do not recommend long-term fasting because of dangers to the kidneys. Short-term fasting is sometimes used by physicians to kick off a diet. The patient foregoes all food under medical supervision, then begins eating small amounts of food while other bodily functions are being carefully monitored.

In recent years the protein-sparing fast has been used for people who have tremendous amounts of weight to lose. That diet includes no solid food but does include certain medications and liquid protein. Protein-sparing fasts should be attempted only under the strict supervision of a physician.

9. Do you think obesity is a symptom of neurosis?

Knowing only that a person is obese is not enough to make a diagnosis. Obesity is no respecter of mental stability. Among the emotionally disturbed, the proportion of thin and heavy people is about the same as that of the general "normal" population. The same is true for intelligence; it is not related to weight.

10. I have lost weight before, but within six months to a year I put it back on again. Any suggestions?

What you are referring to is often known as the "yo-yo" syndrome, that is, weight loss followed by weight gain. It is a common problem for the veteran dieter. What you can learn from this is that you have the capacity to lose weight. That in itself is very encouraging and you should take pride in it. To avoid the weight gain, change your eating patterns, improve your self-talk, maintain good motivation, and generally alter your life-style. By combining the psychological principles presented in this book with a good weight-loss diet, you should be more successful.

11. **I've had a weight-loss problem since adolescence, but it seems more difficult to lose now (in middle age) than when I was younger. Why?**

As we age, our metabolism slows down. This means that we burn fewer calories. Also, age causes our activity level to decline, further reducing the number of calories we burn. Consequently, as we age, it is recommended that we eat less (because we are burning fewer calories) and, when possible, keep up a good exercise or physical-fitness level.

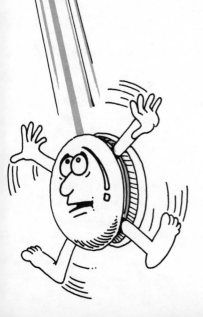

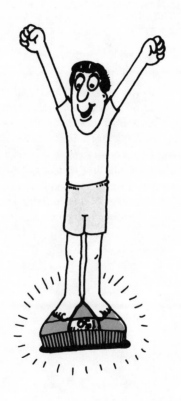

Appendix I Some Special Foods

Special Low-Calorie Foods

These foods are satisfying and contain very few calories. You may eat all you want! Many of them are high in fiber and are especially good for that reason.

beets
broccoli
brussels sprouts
cabbage
cauliflower
celery
cucumbers
green beans
lettuce
mushrooms
onions
radishes
sauerkraut
spinach
unsweetened
  gelatin
watercress

Satisfying Yet Moderate-Calorie Foods

These foods are quite low in calories and are still quite satisfying. Use them to fight off the urge to go on a binge.

apples
apricots
artichokes
asparagus
bread (plain)
cantaloupe
carrots
chestnuts
chicken
cottage cheese
crabmeat
eggplant
fish
grapefruit
lean beef-
  burgers
lobster
mussels
pears
pineapple
  (fresh)
pot cheese
scallops
shrimp
strawberries
tangerines
tomatoes
tuna
turkey

Ultra-High-Calorie Foods

These foods are especially high in calories and are to be avoided at all times.

avocados
baked beans
beer
butter
cake
candy
cheese (in excess)
chocolate
cookies (any kind)
cream and cream substitutes
cream cheese
creamed soups
doughnuts
dressings
dried fruits
duck
fat meats (all kinds)
goose
gravies
ice cream
jams
jellies
macaroni
malted milk
nuts
peanut butter
pie
pizza
pork
soybeans
spaghetti
sugar

Appendix II A Simplified Calorie Chart

Calorie values given for foods in the following tables do not include calories from added fat, sugar, sauce, or dressing—unless such items are included in the listing. Cup measure refers to a standard 8-ounce measuring cup, unless otherwise stated. Foods are listed in the following groups:

- Beverages (carbonated and alcoholic; fruit drinks)
- Bread and cereal group
- Desserts and other sweets
- Fats, oils, and related products (includes salad dressings)
- Meat group (includes fish, eggs, nuts, dry beans and peas)
- Milk group (includes cheeses, milk desserts)
- Snacks and other "extras"
- Soups
- Vegetable-fruit group (includes fruit juices).

BEVERAGES

Calories

Carbonated beverages:
Cola-type	8-ounce glass	95
	12-ounce can or bottle	145
Fruit flavors, 10–13% sugar	8-ounce glass	115
	12-ounce can or bottle	170
Ginger ale	8-ounce glass	75
	12-ounce can or bottle	115
Root beer	8-ounce glass	100
	12-ounce can or bottle	150

(Check the label of "low-calorie" drinks for the number of calories provided.)

Alcoholic beverages:
Beer, 3.6% alcohol	8-ounce glass	100
	12-ounce can or bottle	150

Whiskey, gin, rum, vodka:
80-proof	1½-ounce jigger	95
86-proof	1½-ounce jigger	105
90-proof	1½-ounce jigger	110
100-proof	1½-ounce jigger	125

Wines:
Table wines	3½-ounce glass	85
(Chablis, claret, Rhine wine, sauterne, etc.)		

Dessert wines .... 3½-ounce glass 140
  (muscatel, port, sherry,
    Tokay, etc.)
Fruit drinks:
  Apricot nectar .... ½ cup 70
  Cranberry juice cocktail . . ½ cup 80
  Grape drink .... ½ cup 70
  Lemonade, frozen
    concentrate, sweet-
    ened, ready-to-serve ... ½ cup 55
  Orange juice-apricot
    juice drink. .... ½ cup 60
  Peach nectar .... ½ cup 60
  Pear nectar............... ½ cup 65
  Pineapple juice-
    grapefruit juice drink ... ½ cup 70
  Pineapple juice-
    orange juice drink ..... ½ cup 70

BREAD AND CEREAL GROUP

Bread:
  Cracked wheat .... 1 slice, 18 slices per
                          pound loaf.............. 65
  Raisin................ 1 slice, 18 slices per
                          pound loaf.............. 65
  Rye .... 1 slice, 18 slices per
                          pound loaf.............. 60
White:
  Soft crumb:
    Regular slice .... 1 slice, 18 slices per
                          pound loaf 70
    Thin slice .... 1 slice, 22 slices per
                          pound loaf.............. 55
  Firm crumb............ 1 slice, 20 slices per
                          pound loaf.............. 65
Whole wheat:
  Soft crumb .... 1 slice, 16 slices per
                          pound loaf................65
  Firm crumb............ 1 slice, 18 slices per
                          pound loaf................60
Biscuits, muffins, rolls:
  Baking powder
    biscuit:
    Home recipe .... 2-inch-diameter biscuit.... 105
    Mix .... 2-inch-diameter biscuit.... 90
  Muffins:
    Plain................ 3-inch-diameter muffin 120
    Blueberry 2⅜-inch-diameter
                          muffin.................. 110

Bran	2⅝-inch-diameter muffin.	105
Corn	2⅜-inch-diameter muffin.	125

Rolls:

Danish pastry, plain.	4½-inch-diameter	275
Hamburger or frankfurter.	1 roll (16 per pound)	120
Hard, round or rectangular.	1 roll (9 per pound)	155
Plain, pan	1 roll (16 per pound)	85
Sweet, pan	1 roll (11 per pound)	135

Other flour-based foods:

Cakes, cookies, pies ...	(See Desserts.)	

Crackers:

Butter	About 2-inch-diameter cracker.	15
Cheese	About 2-inch-diameter cracker.	15
Graham	Two, 2½ inches square	55
Matzoth	6-inch-diameter piece	80
Oyster	10	35
Pilot	1	75
Rye	Two, 1⅞ x 3½ inches	45
Saltines	Four, 1⅞ inches square....	50

Doughnuts:

Cake-type, plain	3¼-inch-diameter (1½ ounces).	165
Yeast-leavened, raised	3¾-inch-diameter (1½ ounces).	175

Pancakes (griddle cakes):

Wheat (home recipe or mix).	4-inch cake	60
Buckwheat (with buckwheat pan- cake mix).	4-inch cake	55
Pizza, plain cheese	5½-inch sector of 13¾-inch pie.	155

Pretzels:

Dutch, twisted	1	60
Stick	5 regular (3⅛ inches long) or 10 small (2¼ inches long).	10
Spoonbread	½ cup	235
Waffles	7-inch waffle	210

Breakfast cereals:

Bran flakes (40% bran)..	1 ounce (about 4/5 cup) ...	85
Bran flakes with raisins.	1 ounce (about 3/5 cup) ...	80

Corn, puffed,
  presweetened .... 1 ounce (about 1 cup)..... 115
Corn, shredded .... 1 ounce (about 1-1/6 cups). 110
Corn flakes............ 1 ounce (about 1-1/6 cups). 110
Corn flakes,
  sugar-coated .... 1 ounce (about 2/3 cup) ... 110
Farina, cooked,
  quick-cooking .... ¾ cup 80
Oats, puffed .... 1 ounce (about 1-1/6 cups). 115
Oats, puffed,
  sugar-coated. .... 1 ounce (about 4/5 cup) ... 115
Oatmeal or rolled oats,
  cooked. .... ¾ cup 100
Rice flakes .... 1 ounce (about 1 cup)..... 110
Rice, puffed .... 1 ounce (about 2 cups).... 115
Rice, puffed,
  presweetened........ 1 ounce (about 2/3 cup) ... 110
Rice, shredded .... 1 ounce (about 1-1/8 cups). 115
Wheat, puffed .... 1 ounce (about 1⅞ cups)... 105
Wheat, puffed,
  presweetened........ 1 ounce (about 4/5 cup) ... 105
Wheat, rolled, cooked .. ¾ cup 135
Wheat, shredded,
  plain. .... 1 ounce (1 large biscuit
                        or ½ cup bite-size)....... 100
Wheat flakes .... 1 ounce (about 1 cup)..... 100

Other grain products:
Corn grits, degermed,
  cooked. .... ¾ cup 95
Macaroni, cooked:
  Plain .... ¾ cup 115
  With cheese, home
    recipe. .... ½ cup 215
  With cheese, canned . ½ cup 115
Noodles, cooked....... ¾ cup 150
Rice, cooked, instant... ¾ cup 135
Spaghetti, cooked:
  Plain .... ¾ cup 115
  In tomato sauce,
    with cheese, home
    recipe. .... ¾ cup 195
  In tomato sauce,
    with cheese,
    canned. .... ¾ cup 140
  With meat balls.
    home recipe. ...... ¾ cup 250
  With meat balls,
    canned. .... ¾ cup 195
Wheat germ, toasted ... 1 tablespoon 25

DESSERTS AND OTHER SWEETS

Calories

Cakes:
  Angelcake............... 2½-inch sector of 9¾-
                          inch round cake......... 135
  Boston cream pie .... 2⅛-inch sector of 8-inch
                          round cake. 210
  Chocolate cake, with
    chocolate icing .... 1¾-inch sector of 9-inch
                          round layer cake. 235
  Fruitcake, dark .... 2 x 1½ x ¼-inch slice 55
  Gingerbread............. 2¾ x 2¾ x 1⅜-inch slice ... 175
  Plain cake:
    Without icing .... 3 x 3 x 2-inch slice 315
                          2¾-inch-diameter cupcake. 115
    With chocolate icing ... 1¾-inch sector of 9-inch
                          round layer cake. 240
                          2¾-inch-diameter cupcake. 170
  Pound cake, old
    fashioned .... 3½ x 3 x ½-inch slice 140
  Sponge cake .... 1⅞-inch sector of 9¾-inch
                          round cake. 145

Candies:
  Caramels................ 3 medium (1 ounce)....... 115
  Chocolate creams .... 2 to 3 pieces (1 ounce),
                          35 to a pound. 125
  Chocolate, milk,
    sweetened............. 1-ounce bar 145
  Chocolate, milk,
    sweetened, with
    almonds............... 1-ounce bar 150
  Chocolate mints .... 1 to 2 mints (1 ounce),
                          20 to a pound. 115
  Fondant:
    Candy corn .... 20 pieces (1 ounce) 105
    Mints .... Three 1½-inch mints
                          (1 ounce). 105
  Fudge, vanilla or chocolate:
    Plain................. 1 ounce 115
                          1-inch cube 85
    With nuts............. 1 ounce 120
                          1-inch cube 90
  Gumdrops .... About 2½ large or
                          20 small (1 ounce)....... 100
  Hard candy............. Three or four ¾-inch-
                          diameter candy balls
                          (1 ounce). 110
  Jellybeans .... 10 (1 ounce)............. 105

195

Marshmallows .... 4 large 90
Peanut brittle .... 1½ pieces, 2½ x 1¼ x
                          ⅜-inch (1 ounce). 120

Other sweets:
  Chocolate:
    Bittersweet .... 1-ounce square 135
    Semisweet .... 1-ounce square 145
  Chocolate syrup:
    Thin type............ 1 tablespoon 45
    Fudge type .... 1 tablespoon 60
  Cranberry sauce, canned . 1 tablespoon 25
  Honey .... 1 tablespoon 65
  Jam, preserves .... 1 tablespoon 55
  Jelly, marmalade........ 1 tablespoon 50
  Molasses .... 1 tablespoon 50
  Syrup, table blends ...... 1 tablespoon 55
  Sugar, white, granulated,
    or brown (packed)...... 1 teaspoon 15

Cookies:
  Chocolate chip .... 2-1/3-inch cookie,
                           ½-inch thick 50
  Figbar .... 1 small 50
  Sandwich, chocolate
    or vanilla .... 1¾-inch cookie,
                           ⅜-inch thick 50
  Sugar.................. 2¼-inch cookie 35
  Vanilla wafer .... 1¾-inch cookie 20

Pies:
  Apple .... ⅛ of 9-inch pie........... 300
  Blueberry .... ⅛ of 9-inch pie........... 285
  Cherry .... ⅛ of 9-inch pie........... 310
  Chocolate meringue ..... ⅛ of 9-inch pie........... 285
  Coconut custard........ ⅛ of 9-inch pie........... 270
  Custard, plain .... ⅛ of 9-inch pie........... 250
  Lemon meringue .... ⅛ of 9-inch pie........... 270
  Mince.................. ⅛ of 9-inch pie........... 320
  Peach.................. ⅛ of 9-inch pie........... 300
  Pecan.................. ⅛ of 9-inch pie........... 430
  Pumpkin .... ⅛ of 9-inch pie........... 240
  Raisin.................. ⅛ of 9-inch pie........... 320
  Rhubarb .... ⅛ of 9-inch pie........... 300
  Strawberry .... ⅛ of 9-inch pie........... 185

Other desserts:
  Apple betty............. ½ cup 160
  Bread pudding, with
    raisins .... ½ cup 250

Brownie, with nuts	1¾ inches square, ⅞-inch thick	90
Custard, baked	½ cup	150
Fruit ice	½ cup	125
Gelatin:		
Plain	½ cup	70
With fruit	½ cup	80
Ice cream, plain:		
Regular (about 10% fat)	½ cup	130
Rich (about 16% fat) . . .	½ cup	165
Ice milk:		
Hardened	½ cup	100
Soft serve	½ cup	135
Prune whip	½ cup	70
Puddings:		
Cornstarch, vanilla	½ cup	140
Chocolate, from a mix . .	½ cup	160
Rennet desserts, ready-to-serve.	½ cup	115
Tapioca cream	½ cup	110
Sherbet	½ cup	130

FATS, OILS, AND RELATED PRODUCTS

Butter or margarine	1 pat, 1 inch square, 1/3-inch thick	35
	1 tablespoon	100
Margarine, whipped	1 pat, 1¼ inches square, 1/3-inch thick	25
	1 tablespoon	70
Cooking fats:		
Lard	1 tablespoon	115
Vegetable	1 tablespoon	110
Peanut butter	(See Meat Group; other high-protein foods.)	
Salad dressings:		
Regular:		
Blue cheese	1 tablespoon	75
French	1 tablespoon	65
Home-cooked, boiled . .	1 tablespoon	25
Italian	1 tablespoon	85
Mayonnaise	1 tablespoon	100
Salad dressing, commercial, plain (mayonnaise-type). . .	1 tablespoon	65
Russian	1 tablespoon	75
Thousand Island	1 tablespoon	80

Low calorie:
```
    French ................1 tablespoon .............   15
    Italian................1 tablespoon .............   10
    Thousand Island.......1 tablespoon .............   25
Salad oil .................1 tablespoon ............. 120
```

MEAT GROUP

Calories

Beef:
```
  Beef and vegetable stew:
    Canned ...............1 cup ...................  195
    Homemade, with
      lean beef ...........1 cup ...................  220
  Beef potpie, home
    prepared, baked........ ¼ of 9-inch-diameter pie ..  385
  Chili con carne, canned:
    With beans ...........½ cup ...................  170
    Without beans .........½ cup ...................  240
  Corned beef, canned.....3 ounces ................  185
  Corned beef hash........2/5 cup (3 ounces)........  155
  Dried beef, chipped ......1/3 cup (2 ounces).......  115
  Dried beef, creamed .....½ cup ...................  190
  Hamburger, broiled,
      panbroiled, or
      sauteed:
    Regular ...............3 ounces .................  245
    Lean ..................3 ounces .................  185
  Oven roast, cooked, without bone:
  (Cuts relatively fat, such as rib)
    Lean and fat...........3 ounces .................  375
    Lean only .............3 ounces .................  205
  (Cuts relatively lean, such as round)
    Lean and fat...........3 ounces .................  220
    Lean only .............3 ounces .................  160
  Pot roast, cooked,
      braised or simmered,
      without bone:
    Lean and fat...........3 ounces .................  245
    Lean only .............3 ounces .................  165
  Steak, broiled, without
      bone:
  (Cuts relatively fat, such as sirloin)
    Lean and fat...........3 ounces .................  330
    Lean only .............3 ounces .................  175
  (Cuts relatively lean, such as round)
    Lean and fat...........3 ounces .................  220
    Lean only .............3 ounces .................  160
```

Veal cutlet, broiled,
without bone,
trimmed. . . . . .3 ounces 185
Veal roast, cooked,
without bone. . . . . .3 ounces 230
Lamb:
Loin chop, broiled,
without bone:
Lean and fat. . . . . .3 ounces 305
Lean only . . . . .3 ounces 160
Leg, roasted, without
bone:
Lean and fat. . . . . .3 ounces 235
Lean only . . . . .3 ounces 160
Shoulder, roasted,
without bone:
Lean and fat. . . . . .3 ounces 285
Lean only . . . . .3 ounces 175
Pork:
Bacon, broiled or
fried, crisp. . . . . .2 thin slices 60
                               2 medium slices 85
Bacon, Canadian,
cooked. . . . . .One 3⅜ x 3/16-inch slice . . 60
Chop, broiled, without
bone:
Lean and fat. . . . . .3 ounces 335
Lean only . . . . .3 ounces 230
Ham, cured, cooked,
without bone:
Lean and fat. . . . . .3 ounces 245
Lean only . . . . .3 ounces 160
Roast, loin, cooked,
without bone:
Lean and fat. . . . . .3 ounces 310
Lean only . . . . .3 ounces 215
Sausage:
Bologna. . . . . .2 ounces (2 very thin
                               4½-inch-diameter slices). 170
Braunschweiger . . . . . . .2 ounces (two 3⅛-inch-
                               diameter slices). 180
Pork sausage:
Link, cooked . . . . .Four 4-inch links
                             · (4 ounces, uncooked). . . 250
Bulk, cooked . . . . .Two 3⅞ x ¼-inch patties
                             (4 ounces, uncooked). . . 260
Salami . . . . .2 ounces (two 4½-inch-
                               diameter slices). 175
Vienna sausage,
canned. . . . . .2 ounces (3½ sausages) . . . 135

199

Variety and luncheon
    meats:
  Beef heart, braised,
    trimmed. . . . . .3 ounces (4 x 2½-inch
                       piece). 160
  Beef liver, fried . . . . .3 ounces (6½ x 2⅜ x
                       ⅜-inch piece). 195
  Beef tongue, braised . . .3 ounces (3 x 2 x
                       ⅜-inch piece). 210
  Frankfurter, cooked . . . .1 (8 per pound) 170
  Boiled ham . . . . .2 ounces (2 very thin
                       6¼ x 4-inch slices). 135
  Spiced ham, canned . . .2 ounces (2 thin 3 x
                       2-inch slices). 165

Poultry:
  Chicken:
    Broiled (no skin) . . . . . . .¼ small broiler 115
    Fried . . . . .½ breast 160
                       1 thigh 120
                       1 drumstick 90
    Canned, meat only . . . . .½ cup (3½ ounces) 200
  Poultry pie, home
    prepared, baked. . . . . . .¼ of 9-inch-diameter pie . . 410
  Turkey, roasted (no skin):
    Light meat . . . . .3 ounces 150
    Dark meat . . . . .3 ounces 175

Fish and shellfish:
  Bluefish, baked . . . . .3 ounces (3½ x 2 x ½-
                       inch piece). 135
  Clams, shelled:
    Canned . . . . .3 medium clams and
                       juice (3 ounces). 45
    Raw, meat only . . . . .4 medium (3 ounces). 65
  Crabmeat, canned or
    cooked. . . . . .½ cup (3 ounces) 80
  Fish sticks, breaded,
    cooked, frozen. . . . . . . .Three 4 x 1 x ½-inch
                       sticks (3 ounces) 150
  Haddock, breaded,
    fried. . . . . .3 ounces (4 x 2½ x ½-
                       inch fillet). 140
  Mackerel:
    Broiled with fat . . . . .3 ounces (4 x 3 x ½-
                       inch piece.) 200
    Canned . . . . .2/5 cup with liquid
                       (3 ounces). 155
  Ocean perch, breaded,
    fried. . . . . .3 ounces (4 x 2½ x ½-
                       inch piece). 195

Oysters, raw, meat
   only. .... ½ cup (6 to 10 medium)....   80
Salmon:
   Broiled or baked .... 3 ounces 155
   Canned, pink .... 3/5 cup with liquid
                       (3 ounces). 120
Sardines, canned in
   oil, drained. .... 7 medium (3 ounces) 170
Shrimp, canned .... 27 medium (3 ounces) 100
Tuna fish, canned in
   oil, drained. .... ½ cup (3 ounces) 170
Eggs:
   Fried in fat .... 1 large 100
   Hard or soft cooked,
     "boiled.". .... 1 large   80
   Omelet, plain .... 1 large egg, milk, and
                       fat for cooking.......... 110
   Poached .... 1 large   80
   Scrambled in fat .... 1 large egg and milk 110
Dry beans and peas:
   Baked beans, canned:
     With pork and
       tomato sauce. .... ½ cup 155
     With pork and
       sweet sauce. .... ½ cup 190
   Limas, cooked .... ½ cup 130
   Red kidney beans,
    canned or cooked. ..... ½ cup, with liquid 110
Nuts:
   Almonds .... 15 (2 tablespoons) 105
   Brazil nuts .... 4–5 large (2 tablespoons).. 115
   Cashews .... 11–12 medium
                    (2 tablespoons) 100
   Coconut, fresh,
     shredded. .... 2 tablespoons   55
   Peanuts .... 2 tablespoons 105
   Peanut butter........... 1 tablespoon   95
   Pecans, halves.......... 10 jumbo or 15 large   95
   Walnuts:
     Black, chopped .... 2 tablespoons 100
     English or Persian ..... 6–7 halves   80
                     2 tablespoons, chopped ... 105

MILK GROUP

Calories

Milk:
   Buttermilk .... 1 cup   90
   Condensed, sweetened,
    undiluted. .... ½ cup 490

Evaporated, undiluted.... ½ cup 175
Partly skimmed, 2% nonfat
  milk solids added. .....1 cup 145
Skim..................1 cup 90
Whole.................1 cup 160
Cream:
  Half-and-half (milk
    and cream). ....1 tablespoon 20
                       1 cup 325
  Heavy, whipping ....1 tablespoon 55
  Light, coffee or table .....1 tablespoon 30
  Light, whipping ....1 tablespoon 45
  Sour ....1 tablespoon 25
  Whipped topping,
    pressurized. ....1 tablespoon 10
Imitation cream products
  (made with vegetable fat):
  Creamers:
    Liquid (frozen) ....1 tablespoon 20
    Powdered ....1 tablespoon 10
  Sour dressing (imitation
    sour cream) made with
    nonfat dry milk.........1 tablespoon 20
  Whipped topping:
    Pressurized ....1 tablespoon 10
    Frozen ....1 tablespoon 10
    Powdered, made with
      whole milk...........1 tablespoon 10
Yogurt:
  Made from partially
    skimmed milk..........1 cup 125
  Made from whole milk....1 cup 150
Milk beverages:
  Chocolate-flavored drink
    made with skim milk
    and 2% added butterfat. 1 cup 190
  Chocolate-flavored drink
    made with whole milk ..1 cup 215
  Chocolate, homemade ...1 cup 240
  Chocolate milkshake.....One 12-ounce container... 515
  Cocoa, homemade.......1 cup 245
  Malted milk.............1 cup 245
Milk desserts:
  Custard, baked ....1 cup 305
  Ice cream:
    Regular (about 10% fat) 1 cup 255
    Rich (about 16% fat) ...1 cup 330
  Ice milk:
    Hardened ....1 cup 200

Soft-serve	1 cup	265
Sherbet	½ cup	130
Cheese:		
American, process	1 ounce	105
	1-inch cube	65
American, process cheese food.	1 tablespoon	45
	1-inch cube	55
American, process cheese spread.	1 tablespoon	40
	1 ounce	80
Blue or Roquefort	1 ounce	105
	1-inch cube	65
Camembert	1 wedge of a 4-ounce package containing 3 wedges	115
Cheddar, natural	1 ounce	115
	1-inch cube	70
	½ cup, grated (2 ounces)	225
Cottage, creamed	2 tablespoons (1 ounce)	30
	1 cup, packed	260
Cottage, uncreamed	2 tablespoons (1 ounce)	20
	1 cup, packed	170
Cream	1 ounce	105
	1-inch cube	60
Parmesan, grated	1 tablespoon	25
	1 ounce	130
Swiss, natural	1 ounce	105
	1-inch cube	55
Swiss, process	1 ounce	100
	1-inch cube	65

SNACKS AND OTHER "EXTRAS"

Bouillon cube	1 cube, ½-inch	5
Cheese sauce (medium white sauce with 2 tablespoons grated cheese per cup).	½ cup	205
Corn chips	1 cup	230
Doughnut:		
Cake-type, plain	3¼-inch diameter (1½ ounces)	165
Yeast-leavened, raised	3¼-inch diameter (1½ ounces)	175
French fries:		
Fresh	Ten 3½ x ¼-inch pieces	215
Frozen	Ten 3½ x ¼-inch pieces	170

Gravy	2 tablespoons	35
Hamburger (with roll)	2-ounce patty (about 6 patties per pound of raw meat)	280
Hot dog (with roll)	1 average	290
Olives:		
Green	5 small or 3 large or 2 giant	15
Ripe	3 small or 2 large	15
Pickles:		
Dill	1¾ x 4-inch pickle	15
Sweet	¾ x 2½-inch pickle	20
Pizza, plain cheese	5-1/3-inch sector of 13¾-inch pie.	155
Popcorn, large-kernel, popped with oil and salt.	1 cup	40
Potato chips	Ten 1¾ x 2½-inch chips.	115
Pretzels:		
Dutch, twisted	1	60
Stick	5 regular (3⅛ inches long) or 10 small (2¼ inches long)	10
Tomato catsup or chili sauce	1 tablespoon	15
White sauce, medium (1 cup milk, 2 tablespoons fat, 2 tablespoons flour)	½ cup	200

SOUPS

[Canned, condensed, prepared with equal
volume of water unless otherwise stated]

		Calories
Bean with pork	1 cup	170
Beef noodle	1 cup	65
Bouillon, broth, or consomme	1 cup	30
Chicken gumbo	1 cup	55
Chicken noodle	1 cup	60
Chicken with rice	1 cup	50
Clam chowder, Manhattan	1 cup	80
Cream of asparagus:		
With water	1 cup	65
With milk	1 cup	145
Cream of chicken:		
With water	1 cup	95
With milk	1 cup	180

Cream of mushroom:
　With water ....1 cup 135
　With milk...............1 cup 215
Minestrone ....1 cup 105
Oyster stew (frozen):
　With water ....1 cup 120
　With milk...............1 cup 200
Pea, split ....1 cup 145
Tomato:
　With water ....1 cup 90
　With milk...............1 cup 170
Vegetable with beef broth ..1 cup 80

VEGETABLE-FRUIT GROUP

[Good sources of vitamin C are marked (CC),
fair sources are marked (C), and
good sources of vitamin A are marked (A)]

Calories

Vegetables (raw):
　Cabbage (C):
　　Plain ....½ cup, shredded,
　　　　　　　　　　　　chopped, or sliced 10
　　Coleslaw, with
　　　mayonnaise..........½ cup 85
　　Coleslaw, with
　　　mayonnaise-type
　　　salad dressing. ......½ cup 60
　Carrots (A) ....7½ x 1⅛-inch carrot 30
　　　　　　　　　　　　½ cup, grated............ 25
　Celery ....Three 5-inch stalks 10
　Chicory ....½ cup, ½-inch pieces...... 5
　Chives ....1 tablespoon ....Trace
　Cucumbers, pared ....6 center slices, ⅛-inch
　　　　　　　　　　　　thick 5
　Endive ....½ cup, small pieces 5
　Lettuce ....2 large leaves............ 5
　　　　　　　　　　　　½ cup, shredded or
　　　　　　　　　　　　chopped................. 5
　　　　　　　　　　　　1 wedge, 1/6 of head 10
　Onions:
　　Young green...........2 medium or 6 small,
　　　　　　　　　　　　without tops 15
　　　　　　　　　　　　1 tablespoon, chopped 5
　　Mature ....1 tablespoon, chopped 5
　Parsley................1 tablespoon, chopped ...Trace

Peppers, green	1 ring, ¼-inch thick	Trace
	1 tablespoon, chopped	Trace
Radishes	5 medium	5
Tomatoes (C)	2-2/5-inch diameter tomato	20
Turnips	½ cup, cubed or sliced	20
Watercress	10 sprigs	5

Vegetables (cooked, canned, or frozen):

Asparagus spears (C)	6 medium or ½ cup cut	20
Beans:		
Green lima	½ cup	90
Snap, green, wax or yellow	½ cup	15
Beets	½ cup, diced, sliced, or small whole	30
Beet greens (A)	½ cup	15
Broccoli (A,CC)	½ cup chopped, or three 4½- to 5-inch stalks	25
Brussels sprouts (CC)	½ cup (four 1¼- to 1½-inch sprouts)	25
Cabbage (C)	½ cup	15
Carrots (A)	1 cup	25
Cauliflower (C)	1 cup flower buds	15
Celery	½ cup, diced	10
Chard (A)	½ cup	15
Collards (A, C)	½ cup	25
Corn:		
On cob	One 5-inch ear	70
Kernels, drained	½ cup	70
Cream-style	½ cup	105
Cress, garden (A, C)	½ cup	15
Dandelion greens (A)	½ cup	15
Eggplant	½ cup, diced	20
Kale (A. C)	½ cup	20
Kohlrabi (C)	½ cup	20
Mushrooms, canned	½ cup	20
Mustard greens (A, C)	½ cup	15
Okra	½ cup, cuts and pods	35
	½ cup, sliced	25
Onions, mature	½ cup	30
Parsnips	½ cup, diced	50
	½ cup, mashed	70
Peas, green	½ cup	65
Peppers, green (CC)	1 medium	15
Potatoes:		
Au gratin	½ cup	180
Baked (C)	2-1/3-inch-diameter, 4¾-inch long potato	145

206

Boiled	2½-inch diameter potato...	90
	½ cup, diced	55
Chips	Ten 1¾ x 2½-inch chips....	115
French fries:		
Fresh	Ten 3½ x ¼-inch pieces....	215
Frozen	Ten 3½ x ¼-inch pieces....	170
Hash-browned	½ cup	175
Mashed:		
Milk added	½ cup	70
Milk and fat added	½ cup	100
Made from granules with		
milk and fat added	½ cup	100
Pan-fried from raw	½ cup	230
Salad:		
Made with cooked salad dressing.	½ cup	125
Made with mayon-naise or French dressing and eggs..	½ cup	180
Scalloped without cheese.	½ cup	125
Sticks	½ cup, pieces ¾ to 2¾ inches long	95
Pumpkin (A)	½ cup	40
Rutabagas (C)	½ cup, sliced or diced	30
Sauerkraut, canned	½ cup	20
Spinach, (A, C)	½ cup	25
Squash:		
Summer	½ cup	15
Winter:		
Baked (A)	½ cup, mashed	65
Boiled (A)	½ cup, mashed	45
Sweet potatoes (A):		
Baked in skin (C)	5 x 2-inch potato	160
Candied	½ potato, 2½ inches long ..	160
Canned	½ cup, mashed	140
Tomatoes (C)	½ cup	30
Tomato juice (C)	½ cup	25
Tomato juice cocktail	½ cup	25
Turnips	½ cup, diced	20
Turnip greens (A, C)	½ cup	15
Vegetable juice cocktail	½ cup	20
Fruits (raw):		
Apples	2¾-inch-diameter apple ...	80
Apricots (A)	3 (about ¼ pound)	55
Avocados:		
California varieties	Half of a 10-ounce avocado	190

Florida varieties	Half of a 16-ounce avocado................	205
Bananas	One 6- to 7-inch banana (about 1/3 pound)	85
	One 8- to 9-inch banana (about 2/5 pound)	100
Berries:		
Blackberries...........	½ cup	40
Blueberries............	½ cup	45
Raspberries, red	½ cup	35
Raspberries, black	½ cup	50
Strawberries (CC)	½ cup	30
Cantaloupe (A, CC)	Half of a 5-inch melon.....	80
Cherries:		
Sour	½ cup	30
Sweet	½ cup	40
Dates, "fresh" and dried, pitted, cut.	½ cup	30
Figs:		
Fresh	3 small	95
Dried	1 large	60
Grapefruit (CC):		
White	Half of a 3¾-inch fruit	45
	½ cup, sections	40
Pink or red	Half of a 3¾-inch fruit	50
Grapes:		
Slip skin (Concord, Delaware, Niagara, etc.)	½ cup	35
Adherent skin (Malaga, Thompson seedless, Flame Tokay, etc............	½ cup	55
Honeydew melon (C)	2 x 7-inch wedge	50
Oranges (CC)	2⅝-inch orange............	65
Peaches................	One 2½-inch peach (about ¼ pound)........	40
	½ cup, sliced	30
Pears	One 3½ x 2½-inch pear....	100
Pineapple	½ cup, diced..............	40
Plums:		
Damson..............	Five 1-inch plums (2 ounces)	35
Japanese..............	One 2⅛-inch plum (about 2½ ounces)	30
Raisins.................	½ cup, packed	240
Tangerines (C)	2⅜-inch tangerine (about ¼ pound)........	40
Watermelon (C)..........	One 2-pound wedge	110

Fruits (cooked, canned,
  or frozen):
  Applesauce:
    Unsweetened.......... ½ cup 50
    Sweetened .... ½ cup 115
  Apricots (A):
    Canned in water .... ½ cup, halves and liquid ... 45
    Canned in heavy syrup . ½ cup, halves and syrup ... 110
    Dried, cooked,
      unsweetened. .... ½ cup, fruit and juice 105

  Berries:
    Blueberries, frozen,
      unsweetened. .... ½ cup 45
    Blueberries, frozen,
      sweetened. .... ½ cup 120
    Raspberries, red,
      frozen, sweetened.... ½ cup 120
    Strawberries, frozen,
      sweetened (CC)...... ½ cup, sliced 140
  Cherries:
    Sour, canned in
      water............... ½ cup 50
    Sweet, canned in
      water............... ½ cup 65
    Sweet, canned in
      syrup............... ½ cup 105
  Figs, canned in
    heavy syrup.......... ½ cup 110
  Fruit cocktail, canned
    in heavy syrup. ...... ½ cup 95

  Grapefruit, canned
    (CC):
    Water pack .... ½ cup 35
    Syrup pack .... ½ cup 90
  Peaches:
    Canned in water .... ½ cup 40
    Canned in heavy
      syrup............... ½ cup 100
    Dried, cooked,
      unsweetened. .... ½ cup 100
    Frozen, sweetened ..... ½ cup 110
  Pears:
    Canned in water .... ½ cup 40
    Canned in heavy
      syrup............... ½ cup 95
  Pineapple, canned:
    Crushed, tidbits or
      chunks, in
      heavy syrup.......... ½ cup 95

209

Sliced, in heavy syrup...............	2 small or 1 large slice and 2 tablespoons juice .	80
Plums, canned in syrup ..	½ cup	105
Prunes, dried, cooked:		
Unsweetened..........	½ cup, fruit and liquid	125
Sweetened	½ cup, fruit and liquid	205
Rhubarb, cooked, sweetened..............	½ cup	190
Fruit juices:		
Apple juice, canned	½ cup	60
Grape:		
Bottled................	½ cup	85
Frozen, diluted	½ cup	65
Grapefruit (CC):		
Fresh	½ cup	50
Canned:		
Unsweetened........	½ cup	50
Sweetened	½ cup	65
Frozen concentrate, ready-to-serve:		
Unsweetened........	½ cup	50
Sweetened	½ cup	60
Lemon, raw or canned ...	1 tablespoon	5
Orange (CC):		
Fresh	½ cup	55
Canned, unsweetened..	½ cup	60
Frozen concentrate, ready-to-serve.	½ cup	55
Pineapple, canned, unsweetened.	½ cup	70
Prune, canned...........	½ cup	100
Tangerine, canned (C):		
Unsweetened..........	½ cup	55
Sweetened	½ cup	60

Sun dried - Tomato

1 - 900786-6666

210

Appendix III
A—Daily Calorie-Consumption Record——

Beginning Date_____

Goal for These Two Weeks _____

**Calories
Consumed**

Calories								
3,000								
2,800								
2,600								
2,400								
2,200								
2,000								
1,800								
1,600								
1,400								
1,200								
1,000								
800								
600								
400								
200								
FAST								

Day   1   2   4   6   8   10   12   14

Appendix IV
A—WEEKLY WEIGHT-LOSS RECORD——

First Week_____

Beginning Weight_____

My Weekly Goal Is _____

Pounds Lost

Pounds Lost																
0																
1																
2																
3																
4																
5																
6																
7																
8																
9																
10																
11																
12																
13																
14																
15																
16																

Week 1 2 3 4 5 6 7 8 9 10 11 12 13 14 15 16

BIBLIOGRAPHY

Benson, H. *The Relaxation Response.* New York: Avon, 1976. The author describes how to relax and lists the healthful benefits that accompany learning how to rid ourselves of tension and stress.

Berland, Theodore. *New Ways to Lose Weight . . . Rating the Diets.* Skokie, Ill.: *Consumer Guide,* 1976. This book gives the pros and cons of a large number of diets. The descriptions are clear and concise—an excellent starting point when looking at diets.

Cooper, K. *The New Aerobics.* New York: Bantam, 1970. A book on how to begin a scientific exercise program, how much exercise is enough, and what benefits can be derived from numerous types of physical activity.

Dufty, W. *Sugar Blues.* New York: Warner, 1976. The author presents a historical-to-contemporary use of sugar in our diets and indicates the health problems associated with high sugar intake. Of special note to dieters is his conclusion that large intakes of sugar will increase appetite and hunger.

Ellis, A., and Harper, R. A. *A Guide to Rational Living.* Hollywood, Calif.: Wilshire Book Co., 1968. The authors discuss the link between feelings and thoughts, ways to think ourselves out of emotional upsets, and how to accept reality, control our own destinies, become creative, and live rationally.

Fanburg, W., and Snyder, B. *How to Be a Winner at the Weight Loss Game.* New York: Ballantine, 1975. A behavior-modification book set up to help the reader accurately record food consumption and analyze what occurs concurrently with eating. Helpful ideas are offered about learning to eat more slowly, avoiding distractions that lead to overeating, and becoming aware of "influencers" upon eating, such as feelings, places, and people.

Greenwald, J. *Be the Person You Were Meant to Be.* New York: Dell, 1973. The author distinguishes between "nourishing" and "toxic" living and helps the reader develop antidotes to types of self-induced toxic situations, such as loneliness.

James, M., and Jongeward, D. *Born to Win.* Reading, Mass.: Addison-Wesley, 1971. Very good treatment and application of Transactional Analysis for personal self-understanding. Especially useful for many overweight individuals is the section on "The Drama of Life Scripts."

Leonard, Jon N.; Hofer, J. L.; and Pritikin, N. *Live Longer Now.* New York: Grosset & Dunlap, 1974. This book has excellent chapters on the relationship of diet to degenerative diseases. It shows how to develop an exercise program and introduces the concept of "roving."

McMullin, R. E., and Casy, W. W. *Talk Sense to Yourself.* Denver: Jefferson County Mental Health Center, 1977. This book gives a basic outline for cognitive restructuring. Its aim is to help the reader quickly identify and overcome irrational thoughts with positive self-knowledge.

Maultsby, M. D., and Hendricks, A. *You and Your Emotions.* Lexington, Ky.: Univ. of Kentucky Medical Center, 1974. The authors provide cartoon illustrations of the basic emotional self-help principles and techniques used to help people clean up their "internal dialogues." The book offers pleasant insights into our unwanted emotions and shows what we can do to change them.

Mayer, J. *A Diet for Living*. New York: Pocket Books, 1977. A book that thoroughly covers nutrition, that is, proteins, fats, carbohydrates, vitamins, and minerals. The author recommends a nutritionally sound lifelong diet from toddlerhood to old age. He relates weight to well-being through proper eating and exercise. Helpful ideas on buying and preparing foods are also given.

———. *Overweight: Causes, Cost, and Control*. Englewood Cliffs, N.J.: Prentice-Hall, 1968. The author covers the topics of hunger, obesity, and disease. He discusses genetics and obesity, activity and weight control, social attitudes regarding overweight, the psychology of obesity, and science and nutrition.

Morehouse, Laurence E. *Total Fitness in 30 Minutes a Week*. New York: Pocket Books, 1976. An excellent treatment of the problems of building an exercise program by the man who devised the exercise program for NASA.

Phillips, P., and Cordell, F. *Am I OK?* Niles, Ill.: Argus Communications, 1975. The authors focus on people's OK-ness by facilitating the readers' awareness of each person's inherent potential. They help the reader understand how to move in a positive direction by looking at how to use time, relate to others, and contribute to the well-being of self and others.

Powell, J. *Fully Human, Fully Alive*. Niles, Ill.: Argus Communications, 1976. A very readable book about how our "vision" shapes our lives. The author talks about common misconceptions and the sources that create our perceptions of ourselves, others, and the world around us. A key point throughout the book is that improving our self-talk leads to being "fully human, fully alive."

Robbins, J., and Fisher, D. *How to Make and Break Habits.* New York: Dell, 1976. The authors describe behavior modification and help the reader apply it to breaking habits, including the habit of overeating.

Smith, M. J. *When I Say No, I Feel Guilty.* New York: Bantam, 1975. The author deals with the idea of assertiveness in clear and lucid prose. He outlines a number of assertive skills and shows, through sample dialogues, how they are applied.

Stuart, R., and Davis, B. *Slim Chance in a Fat World.* Condensed ed. Champaign, Ill.: Research Press, 1972. A book on behavioral control of obesity. The authors draw heavily from behavior modification to help the reader design a good weight-control program. They cover nutrition, exercise, and behavioral control of eating habits.

Drs. Cordell and Giebler hold workshops on the psychology of weight loss in several cities. If you would like to be on the mailing list for workshop information, send your name and address to:
The Center for Personal Growth, 2239 12th Street, Greeley, Colorado 80631.